Secrets of Reflex-Crafting

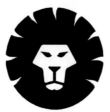

Secrets of Reflex-Crafting

The Cause, Prevention and Treatment of Muscle Pain & Cloaked Muscle Syndrome

By
Sam Craft & Walt Morgan

Editor, Mary Lee Morgan

Colt-Almy Publishing
1000 Little Morro Creek Road
Morro Bay, California 93442

Secrets of Reflex-Crafting
A Colt-Almy Book / April 2002
All rights reserved.

Corel Corporation, graphics
Lippincott Williams & Wilkins; Techpool Studios Inc., medical art
For Information: Reflex-Crafting at
 P.O. Box 6676, Los Osos, California 93412

Library of Congress Cataloging-in-Publication Data
Morgan, Walter S., Craft, Samuel
Secrets of Reflex-Crafting / Walter S. Morgan / Samuel Craft
Library of Congress Control Number: 2002090775
ISBN 0-9709379-0-3
1. Alternative Medicine 2. Massage 3. Holistic Health
1. Secrets of Reflex-Crafting
© 2002

Colt-Almy books are published by Colt-Almy Publishing. Its trademark, consisting of the words "Colt-Almy" and the portrayal of a Colt, is registered in the U. S. Patent and Trademark office and in other countries.
Colt-Almy Publishing, 1000 Little Morro Creek Road, Morro Bay, California 93442

Printed in the United States of America
by Morris Publishing

Dedicated to my sister, who endured
many hardships to put me through
massage school.

...Sam Craft

Dedicated to my mother,
who shared her love of knowledge with
all her children.
...Walt Morgan

Assumptions for the Success of Self-Reflex-Crafting

We are assuming that you can feel pain in the muscle of your body that needs releasing and in your feet and hands. We are assuming that you can bear some discomfort.

We are assuming that you can detect shades of pain rated on a scale from 1 to 10. A No. 1 rating is when a housefly lands on your skin, and No. 10 is pain that hurts so badly that you can't tolerate it. You want to RC Crush starting at level 1 and slowly add pressure until level 7 pain is reached. If you have chronic pain where you need fast relief so that you can get back to work, then push yourself to level 8. Too much pressure at No. 8 can make you sick to your stomach, so use it with moderation. Some people can't tolerate more than level 4 pain. For them, the **Sedative** techniques can work just as well but may take longer to release the muscle. If your back pain does not ease after a sedative treatment, see a doctor.

If you are helping someone else apply RC pain-relief techniques, always remember never to take any person beyond their pain level threshold.

Table of Contents

Table of Contents

Disclosure

Always consult your physician before applying any of these techniques. Do not use Reflex-Crafting techniques if you have the following conditions: diabetes, phlebitis, cardiac problems, blood clotting, acute or unstable infections, fever, disease, acute inflammations of lymphatic and nervous systems, deep vein thrombosis, osteoporosis, decalcification, gangrene or when unstable or risky pregnancy might exist. It is always wise to get a second medical opinion.

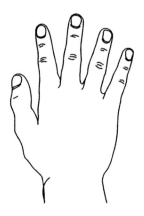

The Power of Touch
Transcends Words

Introduction

The Reflex-Crafting pain relief techniques in this book are powerful tools to help you relieve your pain and to re-establish a clear energy pathway from your brain to the affected pain-causing muscles and tissues in your body.

We have simplified our technique procedures to make them conform to the needs of you, the reader, who is most likely reading this book for self-help. These Reflex-Crafting techniques should be used only when they cannot harm the reader or others. It is not our intention to mislead the reader into believing that Reflex-Crafting is a cure or a substitute for medical treatment or surgery when a doctor recommends either. Our intention is to help the reader understand pain, relieve pain and to regain the mobility of the muscles in his or her body.

We further believe, given the right set of circumstances, that the human body heals itself, so we offer the techniques in this book as a self-help, low-cost alternative procedure that may work to stop pain after modern medical treatments have failed to give relief.

Dr. Fitzgerald's 1916 -1917 Zone Paths through the Hand and Body

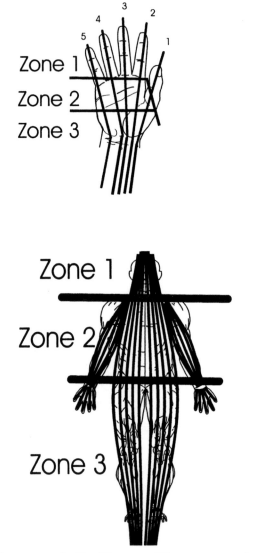

Zone 1

Zone 2

Zone 3

Fitzgerald's Zone Therapy Map

Brief History

Surgeon William Fitzgerald discovered Zone Therapy in 1913. Dr. Fitzgerald developed a Reflex Zone map that divided the human body horizontally into three sections and vertically into ten paths. Each path passed through a toe up to the head and down to a finger. This made a grid map on the body that he separated into three zones. Reflex areas on the hands and feet correlate with these zones.

He discovered that a person could put pressure on an area on the foot or hand and cause a positive response along that entire zone running the length of the body.
Dr. Fitzgerald proclaimed to the medical profession that the body is a wonder of self-healing and self-containment that can benefit from the manipulation of the hands and feet.

From the beginning, Dr. Fitzgerald's work focused on what he and his fellow doctors practiced: nose and oral surgery and dentistry. Most attempts by these pioneers of zone therapy were successful at total pain relief. They found that they could deaden pain and perform surgical operations using this new zone "anesthesia" technique.

By the mid-1920s, the doctors that practiced and taught zone therapy found that they could not afford to spend the necessary time with their patients that the zone treatments required. Thus, there was little or no demand for training doctors or medical students about the techniques of zone therapy. To make zone therapy monetarily acceptable to doctors, zone therapy was reduced to an abbreviated form. This watered-down form made it impractical for use in pain prevention, as it was unreliable in medical situations. With the introduction of pain-relieving medicines that mask pain, the medical establishment quickly abandoned all zone therapy techniques, as drugs offered the "quick fix" for relieving pain that better suited their procedures.

A decade later, under the threat of prison for practicing medicine without a license, alternative medicine advocates fought to take zone therapy methods out of the hands of the medical establishment and to bring the techniques of zone therapy to the layperson.

Building on Dr. Fitzgerald's work, laypersons in the 1930s systemized the reflex areas on the feet and hands in an effort to bring about a normal state in the internal organs and systems of the body. For legal

4

reasons they dropped the medical name "zone therapy" so they could place the emphasis on the overlapping areas of the hands and feet that represented the organs of the body. Any emphasis on pain relief and anesthesia was curtailed so that there would be no appearance of practicing medicine. The new name for this revised therapy in the United States was Reflexology.

Today, most reflexologists use the same or slightly modified techniques developed between 1930 and 1954. They concentrate on the respiratory, endocrine, urinary, reproductive, circulatory, immune and digestive systems where their techniques can specifically address problems related to these bodily systems.

Modern reflexology techniques for pain relief in the musculoskeletal system are generalized. Most reflexology books have little or nothing to say about muscle and fascia tissue pain. They usually show charts that outline a broad area for treating the "back" or the "shoulder" or the "neck." There are no maps or charts that outline the treatment of specific muscles or nerve abnormalities. While present day reflexology and massage will relieve muscle pain, neither has as its sole focus muscle pain relief or muscle renewal.

Today, because of the lifetime work of Sam Craft, an advanced and innovative system for the treatment of the musculoskeletal system has been developed. Using the techniques in this book, anyone can identify reflex points in the feet and/or the hands that can release and sedate specific muscles.

Like Dr. Fitzgerald's initial work on medical anesthesia, Sam Craft's work is a powerful way to interface with the structural muscles and soft tissues of the body and to relieve pain and renew movement. This new therapy is called Reflex-Crafting^{SM}. It is an evolutionary progression from zone therapy.

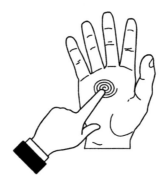

About Sam Craft

Reflex-Crafting was born in the world of horse racing, where men the size of small boys ride in a painful position on fleet-footed, headstrong, masses of moving muscle: the thoroughbred horse. The money is fast, and to win it, the jockey must be fit. Pound for pound, the jockey is the strongest athlete in the world. If he is hurt, he can't ride; if he can't ride, he can't win.

In the spring of 1979, Sam Craft, acting in the capacity as the Official Masseur for professional jockeys at Bay Meadows and Golden Gate Fields Race Tracks in California, had one job to do and very little time to do it in. He had to get these men pain-free and ready to ride before each race. To do this, he needed to push beyond what was known at that time about muscle pain relief. Using all his knowledge as a sixth-degree black belt about how to weaken and destroy the muscles in the human body, he asked himself: Could he use this knowledge in reverse, to help the muscles, so these jockeys could ride pain-free?

Day after day, using himself as a guinea pig, he developed the proven techniques that are shown to you in this book.

A short time after discovering Reflex-Crafting, Sam put his knowledge to work helping jockeys to win their battle against pain and to get back on their horses and race the track. Word got around about his techniques, and when, in 1984, the US Olympic Weight Lifting team needed help, Sam came to their aid. As his success spread, Sam began to get calls from Hollywood celebrities. Stars from television to the big screen needed Reflex-Crafting to get them out of pain and back to work on the set.

Now, because Sam has shared his techniques in this book, anyone can relieve their own pain. He has helped hundreds back to health, from stoke and cerebral palsy victims that could not walk and now do, to breadwinners who were ready to give up their livelihood due to nonstop pain. Sam's work has made many feel that they have found the Fountain of Youth -- or at least feel ten years younger after a treatment!

About Walt Morgan

One day Walt Morgan began experiencing muscle pain problems with his neck from an unknown cause. This pain progressed through the months to a point that, upon waking, he actually felt very little pain at all, but by the afternoon, his pain was so severe that he had to lie down for the rest of the day. He began seeking help through standard medical channels and spent a great deal of money on doctors and tests. X-rays were taken showing no problem. Injections were given but had no effect. Three agonizing years later, after many massage therapist, chiropractor, physiatrist and physician visits, and still suffering with this neck pain that made life and work difficult, with his frustration level at its highest and his spirit at its lowest, a friend suggested that Walt contact Sam Craft, who had helped her with shoulder and arm pain.

Even though skeptical that another professional body worker could do what all the others could not do, Walt contacted Sam for an appointment. After all, he had tried everything he could think of to get pain relief and nothing had worked.

On the day of the appointment, Sam walked in and began his treatment by pressing on Walt's hands. Walt's hopes instantly faded. He thought, "This is going to be another waste of time and money," because he had had reflexology treatments before. However, in less than four minutes, Sam was able to help Walt relieve his pain. Even the large knot on Walt's neck had disappeared.

Then he showed Walt how he could relieve his own pain if it flared up again. It seemed like magic -- it was magic! It was the only treatment Walt ever received from Sam. The three years of misery was over. Walt was so amazed and excited from this miraculous instant relief, he wanted to know more about Sam's treatment and its benefits. He was so enthused that he wanted to share it with others. Walt began studying Eastern and Western massage techniques to learn the basics of massage and reflexology, and was then mentored by Sam to learn Sam's secret pain-relieving techniques. Walt then began exploring the causes of pain and depression and the reasons why Sam's techniques worked far better than other massage or even conventional medical treatments. Calling these techniques Reflex-Crafting, Walt set as his life's mission to get the message out to everyone who suffers from muscle pain that Reflex-Crafting can change their life!

Philosophy of Reflex-Crafting

Reflex-Crafting^{SM}, also known as RC, finds its place in the world of holistic medicine by providing the means for directly addressing the body's structural components -- muscles, joints and nerves -- by working the hands and feet and applying direct pressure on the affected muscle.

To appreciate the philosophy of Reflex-Crafting, one must understand that it is the simplicity of the Reflex-Crafting system that makes it a dynamic body/mind-working tool.

There are only four maneuvers or techniques to be learned by the reader. Most people can produce results with just elementary training. The chances of hurting yourself or someone else when Crafting is rare because of this simplicity. It is applied through an easy-to-follow process outlined in this book. The Reflex-Crafting philosophy is simplicity -- simplicity with dynamic results on the body and mind.

Reflex-Crafting uses pressure on the hands and feet to address the brain so it can release the pain from muscles. Reflex-

Crafting is not reflexology. While reflexology does use the hands and feet, it does so to mainly focus on the body's internal organs. Reflex-Crafting is structural. Reflex-Crafting addresses structural muscles, nerves, fascia, as well as blood chemistry, and the mental and emotional states of the mind/muscle connection, not internal organs nor the other physiological systems.

In this book we will explain how Reflex-Crafting directly addresses your lower brain through your hands and feet; plainly stated, how it speaks directly to the lower brain in the language of the lower brain and how Reflex-Crafting reassigns a hurting muscle by placing that muscle in a higher, healthier position on the lower brain's hierarchical muscle list.

Structurally, Reflex-Crafting uses three horizontal zones and an unlimited number of vertical paths to form micro-zones, which we call the RC grid. The RC grid is not flat but is three-dimensional. It differs also from Dr. Fitzgerald's zone therapy, which the primary use was for anesthesia during nose and throat surgery. Reflex-Crafting works not only on RC points on the hands and feet, but also by applying sedative techniques on the affected structural muscles of the body.

Releasing these affected muscles is a necessary part of the RC treatment.

Treating the structural RC points on the hands and/or feet and then the corresponding tissue or muscles brings about a homeostasis not only to the area being treated but also to the whole body/mind in general. In fact, it causes such positive change to the lower brain that a new mental disposition forms. This peace of mind goes on to reinforce the physical results in following treatments.

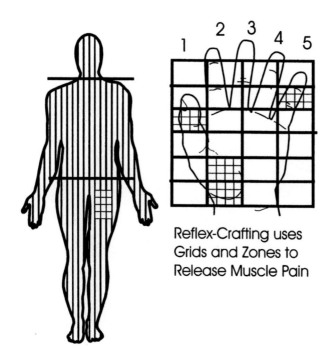

Reflex-Crafting uses Grids and Zones to Release Muscle Pain

How to Use this Book

This book is divided into two parts. The first part of this book is about Reflex-Crafting theory. We address why the brain ignores or strengthens some muscles, as well as why a muscle in the body can silently decline. You should find Reflex-Crafting theory provides you with insight on why your body hurts and what you can do to stop hurting muscles.

Reflex-Crafting theory unlocks for the first time some of the secrets of why we suffer pain and stiffness and why we get depressed or hurtful to others. RC theory brings to light the reasons behind our negative human nature and the major cause of our human condition. It also gives us a clear path to find better health and happiness for ourselves and for everyone around us.

The second part of this book contains simple, straightforward Reflex-Crafting pain-relief techniques. It addresses the use of Reflex-Crafting to relieve physical and emotional pain in the body. Both advanced body workers or novices can use the book's Crafting charts to locate muscles and body areas. In part two of this book, the reader can review examples of how Sam Craft releases the hips and lower back. Each example outlines the steps needed to relieve the pain through the hands and feet and the muscles involved.

Using the four Reflex-Crafting techniques, you and people in pain or under emotional or physical attack can directly appeal to the brain for its help. Once the brain sends this help, pain in the area is either dosed with natural pain relief or, in the best-case scenario, repaired by the body.

As a student of Sam Craft, I have used my study of Reflex-Crafting to attempt to understand and explain the relationship that exists between the human brain and its body. I do this in the hope of helping others live a pain-free life.

Both Sam Craft and I know that you, too, will find Reflex-Crafting eye-opening and life-changing.

Chapter 1

Reflex-Crafting Theory

Reflex-Crafting has the ability to restructure a friendly relationship and renew the partnership between the human brain and the structural muscles of the human body. It is our belief that the brain perceives and works with the human body's muscles using a structural hierarchy list. This muscle hierarchy list is defined in Reflex-Crafting as a muscle priority system, where certain muscles are more or less favored or developed than other muscles by the brain.

This hierarchy of the muscles is easily observed during the transformation of babies into toddlers. As a baby grows, we can see that his muscles develop in a systemized maturation pattern permitting the baby to first stand, then to walk. In normal human development, the brain and the chemistry of the body assigns muscles to take on different physical forms as needed throughout a person's lifetime. This steady muscle transformation can be witnessed as the child matures in both the female and male bodies. As the body grows and matures, different muscles in each sex are developed for a required form and function. In each sex muscles may be at first limited in their strength, endurance and motion, while other muscles in the maturing body are allowed to be well formed and become stronger or more flexible.

It is evident in maturing adults that, over a lifetime, the muscle hierarchy of an individual entitles certain chosen muscles in his or her body to prosper and sentences others to decline and become painful or, worse, to be cloaked. The brain stops using these declined muscles or parts of their muscle fibers to move the body efficiently. The near abandonment of many bundles of muscle fibers by the brain can be observed in some elderly people whose low priority muscles cause their shoulders to slump over and their feet to shuffle as they walk.

Over time, most people experience muscles that are limited in their duties and motion. To date, science has not discovered the overall reasons for the body's muscle hierarchy and why some muscles are limited or why large amounts of muscle fibers are moved to near abandonment by the brain.

They do find evidence on a greater scale of a human organ and muscle hierarchy. In your body, there is an organ that has been abandoned; that organ is your appendix. There is no known use for the appendix but it still exists in your body. Many researchers believe the human appendix will, over time, not exist in the bodies of future humans. There are some that theorize that the entire bone and muscles of the fifth toe (little toe) on the human foot will be absorbed into the fourth toe in later generations of humans. The little toe is not necessary for standing or walking and it is believed to be in the process of being absorbed by the body.

There are signs of total muscle abandonment in humans. The palmaris longus muscle in the arm is missing in some humans. The psoas minor muscle that is used by four-legged animals, can be found in less than half of all humans. Why this muscle exists in some of us and not in others is not known. It may be that muscle, bone and organ abandonment is essential to the final, and yet unknown, evolving form of human beings.

While many researchers believe that evolution is the reason behind muscle, bone and organ abandonment, there is disagreement as to the cause of muscle decline in an individual over his or her lifetime. As practitioners of Reflex-Crafting, we believe it is not a future evolutionary plan for the human body but a prehistoric survival factor that is behind muscle fiber decline in individuals.

In Reflex-Crafting theory, we interpret the health of a muscle according to its position on the brain's Muscle Hierarchy List. This list determines what muscles will be strengthened or decline in each individual and what muscles will experience pain and stiffness.

We believe that in normal healthy human development, beginning as an infant and progressing to maturity, the brain assigns muscles to take on different and needed physical forms. In this process, healthy muscles are strengthened or normalized in an ongoing maturation process following the brain's survival needs. Every muscle is not needed by the brain for you to survive, so muscles are assigned an importance by your brain based on this need to survive. Using its "Muscle Hierarchy List" the brain assigns each muscle in your body a survival ranking. This leads us to believe that when a muscle is not healthy, long after an injury to it has healed, or if pain comes on suddenly with no known cause, then that muscle has lost its position on the brain's hierarchical list . Any muscles that have been assigned to the bottom of the list are not necessary for survival and are listed for future abandonment by the reptilian brain.

Modern science does not know the history of the appendix, nor does it know the history of the toes or tail, as there are no fossil records showing a missing link. Nevertheless, what we can assume is that the brain knows why it chooses certain organs, bones and certain muscles to perform a function and why it chooses to abandon those muscles, bones and organs at a later time.

In this book, we present my theory on muscle hierarchy and Sam Craft's techniques on how to reassign declining muscles a new position on the brain's muscle hierarchy list.

Chapter 2

Understanding the Form and Function of Muscles:

Each animal species has a unique shape or muscle form to its body so that it can act or move within a niche in its supporting environment. It could be said that an animal is a wonderfully designed tube that has adapted itself to live on a water planet. Food and water that enters one end of the tube is converted into energy, then the unused by-products go out the other end of the tube. These tubes fly in the air, swim in the sea, or walk on or burrow in the ground. Tubes called mammals have adapted a vast array of differing exteriors and muscular forms to take advantage of niches in their supporting earthly environments. The form and function of bats, elephants and whales are an example of this ability to vary the mammalian tube. Muscles and tissue make up the exterior form of these three different mammals. Their bones adapted to hold their muscles and tissues in place. The total muscle form of each of these mammals is specifically designed to live or function in either a combination of environments such as water, land or air, or in the case of the whale, a specific environment, water only.

Three Life Forces on Muscles

We understand that life comes from life. No matter what name man gives to a mammalian life form, it did not come into its present state from isolation. It carries information for its survival and body form in its genes.

Reflex-Crafting theory begins with the hypothesis that three major environmental forces form the muscular outward appearance of mammals. The first environmental force on the mammal's form is its supporting environment: air, water or land.

The second environmental force on the mammalian form is the food source or niche from which each animal will receive its life-giving energy. These food niches are made up of energy sources existing in the water, air or on or under the land.

If the food in the energy niche lives under the land, such as ants do, then any mammal that needs to eat from that food niche will find that its body comes under natural forces that will re-form its muscles and tissue into an efficient form for the eating of ants. As it will take many ants to feed a mammal, this force will continue to adapt the mammal's form to the eating of ants until it reaches a point where this animal has reached a positive energy balance. At this point it will stop evolving its muscle form. An ant-eating mammal reaches its peak muscle form when the energy that it uses to exist and produce offspring is less than the energy that it burns finding and eating ants. When that energy balance is reached, scientists call that mammalian muscle form a Myrmecophaga tridactyla or giant anteater.

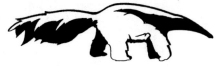

This peaked muscle form has been walking the earth for hundreds of thousands of years unchanged and balanced in its niche.

If the food source for a mammal will be a woolly mammoth, then the muscles and tissues of that mammal will re-form for the hunting and eating of mammoths. Scientists have called the muscle formation that eats woolly mammoths a saber-toothed cat. Again, what they are naming is not an animal but a muscle form that a tube or mammal has adopted so that it can eat a specific food. If a food niche is no longer available, the body form of a mammal will change again to eat from a new source of energy. A mammal's body form may no longer be called an ant-eater or saber-toothed cat, for that mammal may have to change its muscular form so drastically to come into balance with its new form that it is not recognized in its old form. Its new muscular form will change it into a different animal so it can eat from a new energy source efficiently.

We see the form of mammals changed by this force in fossil records. The ancestors of the great whales once walked the land as another muscle form of a mammal that scientists call a Mesonychid. This ancestor of the whale looked like a house cat with a long face. They changed their form over time to seek the food niche of the sea. If today a whale form tries to come back to land and is beached, it will die. Its muscle form can no longer support it as the land mammal it used to be.

The third major force on an animal's muscular form and the functions of their muscles is the animal's position in the food chain. The reality of "Eat and be Eaten" is part of most mammals' daily experience. Animals that prey on the mammal force that mammal to adapt an evasive or other defensive form in order to survive. The horns of the Cape buffalo, the spray of the skunk or the razor-sharp teeth of the hippopotamus all defend their muscle forms from being eaten.

Other animals, such as zebras, rabbits and horses, evade predators by fleeing. The next time you see a horse, look at each part of the horse. Each part of its form contributes to the survival of the horse as an individual and as a species. When you are looking at a horse, you are seeing a mammal that was formed by where it lives and what it eats and by what eats its muscles. Because the horse is hunted, there is no other reason for the horse's body shape or its size, speed, strength and on-edge senses than to protect its muscles from being eaten. What you see when you look at a horse is a muscle form that has come into balance and, for the most part, was created solely to evade and flee a big cat.

When an animal is eaten by a predator, it is not because it is an individual and is being singled out on the menu of life. It is eaten because it is a member of a species that is the energy niche or food source for that predator's peak muscle form. If the predator has not peaked and becomes faster than the prey, then the prey must adapt either to become faster or find another way to counter the speed of the evolving predator. All mammals, including man, must adapt and have adapted their forms to protect themselves as a species from predators. To adapt, a species may get faster, grow larger, climb higher, and add camouflage or produce more offspring than can be taken by the predator so that they can survive as a species. They can also adapt their defensive strategies as to how they are perceived by the predators.

For example, zebras use stripes to lessen their chances of being killed. Stripes do not help a lone zebra survive. Stripes only work as a survival strategy when many zebras are running together.

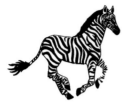

A lone zebra
is easily seen.

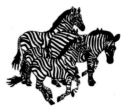

Here a young zebra is protected
by the stripes of the herd.

The stripes confuse the predator as she tries to keep her eye on one particular animal, only to see a moving wall of black-and-white stripes. We can safely state that without the big cat, the zebra would not have black-and-white stripes. This is because the zebra herd's defense strategy depends on the big cats, who only see in black and white, seeing their stripes.

Predators also are forced to adapt. When large prehistoric mammal populations declined, so did the numbers of saber-toothed cats. The saber-toothed cat had formed muscles specifically designed to hunt only large mammals, such as the bison and mammoth. During the decline of these large mammals, this big cat could not adapt its muscle form or its function fast enough to hunt other prey. The saber-tooth could not compete with other meat-eaters who were well adapted for killing food in their own niche. The saber-toothed cat died off because it lacked the adaptability to rebalance its form .

Some predators have adapted specialized sensory organs to help them locate food. For example, the bat, porpoise and the honey badger all use sonar to locate their food in their different supporting environments. The reptilian alligator has nerve endings on both sides of its head that can feel the movement of animals up to three feet away while it is submerged in muddy water. It need not open an eye to locate and snap a meal into its jaws. Another example of a hunter with specialized senses is the sperm whale that projects sound waves from its skull to locate and stun giant squid in the deepest waters of the ocean.

Some carnivores have the ability to sense weak or hurt prey from long distances. The mako shark can sense a distressed animal miles away through its ability to perceive unusual electrical impulses from its prey's muscle contractions. It could be that the reason behind unpredictable shark attacks on humans is linked to the muscle conditions of those people who are attacked.

Humans have no obvious defensive

strategy against attack. Even though we think we can run fast (5 miles an hour), a two-ton elephant (25 miles an hour) can outrun any man. Humans do not use fangs or claws to defend themselves. It would appear that humans could not survive the attack of any large animal that sought to kill us, yet we do survive. We have a hidden defense, and that is our upper brain. While other animals use the instincts of the lower brain to survive, our prehistoric ancestors used the upper brain to learn to hunt by watching animals that hunt and learned to fish from animals that fish, and learned to survive by watching other animals survive.

Today, we humans seldom think about the influences of our lower brain. We live and think as if we only have an upper, well-educated, rational brain. We perceive ourselves only in terms of the modern self. Therefore, most people believe that ancient history ended the day before their grandparents were born. There is little thought given, as each of us looks into the mirror, that what stands naked before us is a human life form that was adapted by what it ate and what ate it.

To understand muscle pain, we need to realize that we live in a muscle form that adapted and balanced itself to survive in the prehistoric environment of 50,000 years ago. Our body has not changed since that time. Even though both the upper brain and the body that we live in today stopped evolving and peaked in its form and function long ago, not a thought of this fact passes through the average person's mind. Most of us view every event in life based on how it affects our modern lifestyle and not what effect each of life's changing events has on our 50,000-year-old brain and its muscles.

Chapter 3

Understanding Your True Self

Many humans want to believe that they are single, self-sufficient, well-educated individuals, living among other individuals that are either less or more self-sufficient and educated than they are. When you view the environment through the eyes of a modern human, this belief could be perceived to be true. However, at a scientific level it is not true, because a true individual, according to scientists, are single animal forms that have little connection to or need for other individuals of their own species.

In lower forms of life, single beings make no contact with each other; they even reproduce asexually. In higher forms, such as apes, the orangutang in the wild lives a solitary life for most of the year, making very brief, one-on-one contact with the opposite sex only during the mating season. This great ape could live its whole adult life in isolation from its own kind and be happy and healthy. The orangutan is a self-sufficient individual; whereas, man is not. We need contact with other humans for our well-being and survival. If we are isolated, we will go mad.

If human life were viewed by little men from Mars, back when the ancestors of humans walked the grasslands of Africa, long before our kind discovered fire, long before we hunted, these Martians would say that we were not a group of individuals living together. They would say that our muscle form and our muscle function at that time resembled more the animals that we traveled with: wild cattle, wildebeests and zebra. They would list us among the many animals in the great migrating herds and not among the carnivores that preyed on the great herds of the African savanna.

Back then, our ancestors traveled with the great herds. To insure that each species that made up the herd had a source of food, each species ate from its own niche. Zebras ate only the coarse grass. Wildebeests ate only the softer grasses. Wild cattle ate only the low grass. Our ancestors ate the tubers, seeds and insects. This way, all the members of the herd were able to survive as they moved across the land. Our ancestors also traveled with the herd for the protection and safety that only a herd can give. But how can this be? Are we not great hunters? Have we not reached the top of the carnivore's food chain? We eat shark. We eat bear. We eat carnivores. Yes, we watched and learned our lessons very well. We are at the top of the food chain, but that does not change the fact that our muscles and tissues are those of a 50,000-year-old gatherer, not those of a hunter.

If we look at the muscles and tissues in mammals that are hunters -- for example, inside the mouth of an African lion -- we see 30 teeth. Every tooth in his mouth has a form and a function. That function is to kill or slice or tear. The muscles in his jaw are also perfect in their form and function. They will drive his fangs through the thick leathery hide of his prey. Remove any of those teeth and you have lessened his chances of survival. Remove his large incisors that he uses to kill and hold his prey with and he will starve to death.

Look into your own mouth. Like the lion, your teeth are in sets. Each tooth has a purpose for being there. They are just the right number, the right size and shape, as are the muscles in your jaw, for you to survive 50,000 years ago. You will notice that your teeth are not at all like the teeth of the flesh-eating lion. Your teeth are not like the teeth of any predator. You might be able to kill a baby bird, but beyond that, your teeth and jaw muscles do not have the right form and function for killing. Human teeth are made for eating fruits, nuts, tubers and soft foods.

Your jaw muscles are still functioning as they did thousands of years ago, and your muscular form is the same as your prehistoric plant-eating mother who gave birth to her likeness, who, in turn, gave birth to her likeness, and so on, until your mother gave birth to you. Same form, same function. Their DNA is your DNA.

What makes us the great meat hunters that we are today? What is sharper than any fang or claw? It is our brain.

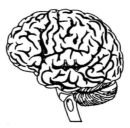

Chapter 4

Your Three Brains

Scientist Dr. Paul MacLean, M.D., a neuroanatomist, theorized in 1975 that our one large brain is actually divided into three different brain functions. Each brain is stacked one on top of the other: the ancient brain, called the reptilian brain; the emotional brain or mammalian limbic brain; and the upper brain, called the rational thinking brain (cerebral cortex).

The ancient brain sits on the top of the spine. This ancient reptilian brain resembles and functions like the brain of the dinosaurs. Sitting on top of this ancient brain is an emotional brain called the limbic system. It is found in other mammals as well. Covering those two brains is a new but much slower brain that is less than two million years old: the rational brain (cerebral cortex). Before any information can reach the newer rational brain, it must pass through filters in the other two older brains. If the reptilian brain senses a perceived threat, the reptilian brain reacts to that threat before any emotions or thinking can take place by the other brains.

Once the reptilian brain processes and relays any orders to the glands or muscles, then that information is passed to the emotional brain. This brain, called the limbic system, filters the information. It colors all messages that pass through it. This coloring is emotional. We laugh and cry because of this brain. This brain will broadly paint any information it receives. If you had an emotional experience, either good or bad, that made you laugh or cry in your past, any like occurrence that is filtered by the mid-brain will be colored with that same emotional response by the mid-brain. Your first emotional experiences are never forgotten, such as your first kiss, your first love or your first major embarrassment. That is why, when talking with a group of people, you may be the only one that laughs or cries or gets angry about the subject under discussion. This happens when your emotional brain filters and then colors the subject that is being talked about.

The cerebral cortex or upper brain is the brain that you are using to try to understand what I am writing. It is the brain where language is formed and it is the brain that tries to control the other two brains. It is the civilized brain. The rational upper brain does not react, it slowly thinks.

The two quick-reacting brains that do not think filter all information that comes from our five senses, then pass it on to the rational brain. This is why the upper brain does its purest work on non-threatening, unemotional subjects, such as math and science. Whenever the upper brain labors on threatening and emotional subjects that have been passed on to it by the other two brains, the information is not pure; it is an afterthought.

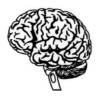

In Charles Darwin's theory of evolution, we read about life evolving from simple forms to complex forms. Darwin might say that man evolved from a small mammal. This evolution was made possible by time, chance and changes to the small mammal's form. If we did evolve from that small mammal, our human brain did not evolve. As Dr. MacLean points out, it just added on new parts to some very old brain parts that the small mammal had. Those old parts have not evolved or changed one bit and they are not going to be changed by thinking, reading or higher education. They are fixed in the past.

To make it easier to understand the brain's parts, think of the lower brain as an old house. This very old house over the years had some major additions built on to it. The original house, with its foundation, was built in 1025 BC out of rock and heavy timbers. It has a large fire pit and very small windows. Much later, in 1813, the second-story children's nursery and mother-in-law's rooms were built above the old house. Last year a third story was built. This is where the entertainment room and library are located, as well as the computer room and music room. Like many homes that have add-ons, there have been many compromises made.   The major complaint of the owner is that visitors must first walk in through the heavy doors of the old house and up the narrow staircase to the second floor. They then are subject to the customs of emotional greetings, handshakes and hugs, as well as the noise of laugher and crying before they can reach the upper level. Only then can they speak on the meaning of life or channel surf the television.

It is our belief in Reflex-Crafting that the old house, called the lower or reptilian brain, perceives and interacts with the muscles and nerves of the human body through a structural form and a functional hierarchy or ranking system. Muscles needed for survival of the brain have a higher priority than muscles that are not needed to survive. This is a totalitarian hierarchy and it is based solely on the reptilian brain's perceived need for the survival of our species. The rational brain and emotional brain have no voice in the decision. All survival threats encountered by the brain are categorized by the reptilian brain. This ranking is based on the brain's perception of its risk of death from the threat. Because humans are raised in different environments, they perceive information differently, causing each human's reptilian brain to react to its risk of death differently. This can cause a back muscle of one person to hold a high ranking on their hierarchy list and the identical back muscle on another person's list to hold a low ranking.

Three people can be walking in the woods and all see the same poisonous snake. One person may run from it, another person may ignore it, and another may kill the snake. We witness in our daily lives different lower brains filtering the same information but having different reactions to the same stimuli. What we cannot see is what muscles the brain uses for its survival purposes when that old brain reacts to a threatening stimulus. Only the ancient brain knows and records this knowledge on its muscle hierarchical list.

Like your muscles, each of your three brains has a form and a function. Dr. Paul MacLean's theory states that there are three different brains controlling three different functions in the human body. The brain that oversees your muscles is the lower brain, which, in his theory is called the reptilian brain. The basic need to survive is under the control of this lower reptilian brain. The parts of this brain are the medulla, pons, cerebellum, mesencephalon, globus pallidus and olfactory bulbs. All these parts are called the "R-complex" by Dr. MacLean. This lower brain does not think. Its function is to react, using a threat hierarchy list as a guide.

A lizard or a snake only has a reptilian brain. They are being governed only by this brain. They do not cry and they do not plan for their future. They just react. Their brain is like an internal clock. The clock goes off with an alarm any time the brain perceives danger.

Your reptilian brain, like the lizard's, has two functions. First, its function is to keep you alive and, secondly, and most importantly, its function is to keep your species alive. To keep you alive, your reptilian brain manages and controls your heartbeat, temperature and breathing. It also manages your muscles without your participation or knowledge for your survival. Many times during the day you will not know whether you are controlling your muscles or if the lower brain is in control. This lower brain-controlled state happens throughout the day for many of us, more often than not when we are eating or walking or driving.

We need and rely on this very old brain. It works day and night without rest to keep us alive. This reptilian brain uses powerful forces to do its work, forces that protect not only ourselves, but also forces that protect our family, our tribe and our life form or species. Our brain forces work together for our benefit and the benefit of our tribe. However, if there is a conflict between the individual force (self) and the other three forces that protect our family, tribe or species, the self or individual force will lose. So, when any of these other forces come into conflict with the force that protects each of us as individuals, we can be overwhelmed by our very own brain with stress. Conflict within an individual's family leads to major stress on the muscles of the body. The brain then attacks the muscles, nerves and skin of the person who is in conflict with the family until that person stops the conflict.

An example of a conflict between the major force of protecting the tribe and protecting yourselves can be seen in times of war when we, as individuals, are sent to risk our lives to protect our tribe by the lower brain. Any that refuse to fight for the tribe are pushed away, and their muscles and nerves may be attacked by the lower brain. As in the

Macbeth passage, "The coward dies many times before his death; The valiant never taste of death but once."

Those that are successful in the risking of their lives for others are made into heroes and legends by the tribe.

Conflicts between the species force and the individual force are revealed by the belief that killing an enemy's children is wrong, that genocide is wrong and that eating other humans is wrong. If we find that individuals have crossed these lines, we, in fact, as a tribe, punish them.

When we are in conflict with groups of people, such as our family or fellow workers, we feel the stress generated by the lower brain. This stress leads to pain. That stress-pain is held in the muscles of our body and gives out an energy signal that can be detected. The more conflict or stress we incur between these old brain forces, the stronger the pain that we have in our bodies.

The reptilian brain has successfully been doing its job to balance its forces so that we survive as individuals, families, tribes and as a species for millions of years. It is not going to change.

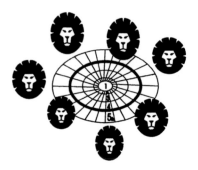

Chapter 5

Survival Strategies

Since the beginning of our time as humans, we have been hunted by big cats that sought out the young, the hurt, the sick and the weakened among us. The reality of being human is to recognize that big cats not only helped form other herd animals, like the zebra, but as a predator of humans, they had a part in determining our muscle form and defining us as a species.

All the carnivores that prey on herd animals, such as lions, leopards and hyenas, consider monkeys, apes, baboons and humans as food. Big cats still hunt us for food. In 2000, tigers killed and ate over 70 of us. In every attack, the human was taken down by a single bite to the right nape of the neck. The big cats instinctively know how to kill the naked ape.

The adult African lion needs to eat eleven to eighteen pounds of flesh every day or 120 lbs. a week. A large pride of lions can eat one or more of our fellow herd animals every day, be it zebras, wildebeests, cattle or humans. It can do this year after year, and their offspring will grow up and continue to do it after they are gone -- eighteen pounds of us each and every day. There are thousands of lions, panthers, and leopards out in the wild and they are all hungry.

Herd animals and big cats have lived together for thousands of years. All herd animals instinctively know that the lions must eat. They know and fear that the lions will kill one of them that day, and another one of them the next day, and the next and the next.

Millions of years before man, plant-eating dinosaurs with reptilian brains walked the earth, eating its flora. Unlike the reptiles that we see today, their reptilian brains required them to form herds. Modern plant-eating mammals, with their dinosaur-like reptilian lower brains, still form herds. One would think that the purpose of a plant-eating mammal, like man, to form a tribe, or for mammals to gather into herds of thousands, is for the protection of the individuals in that herd or tribe. It makes sense that any individual that is being hunted would seek the safety of numbers. But, as stated previously, we herd animals are not individuals. Therefore, Reflex-Crafting theory concludes that this is not the reason herds are formed.

The function and form of a herd is for the protection of the species from predators, not the protection of all of its individual members. Thousands of years ago, our ancestors joined these herd animals to form a large migrating herd. By joining as members of the great herd, our ancestors added to the herd's defenses eyes that could see the color and shape of a lion in the dry golden grass and the ability to communicate a warning to all members of the herd. This added another layer of protection to the herd and protected each species' young and pregnant females from being taken and eaten by big cats and other predators.

Some examples of big cats are lions,

panthers, jaguars, tigers and several species of extinct cats. These big cats have adapted survival strategies to counter the herd's defenses. A female cat with cubs risks her life and their lives each time she hunts. She finds it dangerous, if not deadly, to attack a herd of healthy, kicking and goring animals. A lion will sleep eighteen hours a day just to build up the energy that it takes to hunt. Each time she hunts and fails to take an animal, she puts her family's life at risk by wasting this reserve energy. This in turn weakens the cat and makes her less likely to make a kill after each failed attempt on healthy animals. To stay strong and to keep from being gored or having her jaw kicked off, the big cat must be very cautious about what animal it chooses to attack.

To stay out of danger, we believe that big cats evolved a sixth sense, such as the mako shark has done, that detects weakness in the muscles of their prey. This is a sense like smell and sight; it provides the cat with the ability to locate specific weakened animals in a herd of thousands of healthy, kicking and goring animals. The big cats use this sixth sense to detect weakness in the herd animals before she makes any attempt to attack them.

In order to protect their species from becoming extinct, herds must guard their young and their healthy fertile females from attack.

It is thought that some extinct big cats had, and that the African lion of today has, the ability to receive and read energy waves sent out from the herd animals she hunts that tells her the physical health and condition of those animals. Using this sense, the big cat can locate a few animals in a herd of hundreds that are suffering sore, torn, tired or weakened muscles from an astounding 200 feet away.

These muscle-sensing big cats hunt mostly at night. Night hunting is dangerous for the big cat. While these big cats have excellent night vision, their night vision is limited. They cannot see the strength or read the body language of their prey at night. An unseen kick from an aggressive bull or pro-tective mother can break a tooth or a jaw or crack a skull. Any injury can lead to the big cat's death. When hunting, lions use this special muscle sensing to select the weakest, most easily killed animals from among the stronger and life-threatening animals in the herd. In the pitch-blackness of the night, this ability to sense weakness protects her from the risk of injury and death before she makes her attack.

We know that most animals have an obvious defense against predators. It may be running, flying, chemical spray, or it may be a fang, claw, hoof or horn. Less obvious is the defenses that predators have against their prey. Even the great white shark, the killing machine of the seas, closes its eyes just before it bites. Then it runs off and lets the prey bleed and weaken before returning to eat. Reading muscle signals of animals is the lion's defense against its prey, because there is no safe large prey that can be taken without risk to her life. In fact, it is known that Cape buffalo bulls will stalk and hunt for lions at night, hoping to kill them by using their horns and hooves.

Defense Strategies of the Herd

To protect the young and healthy fertile females, different species of animals adapted defensive strategies. One of the most successful strategies is the tribe or herd itself with hundreds of eyes, ears and noses to detect a threat. The herd strategy has many elements within it to protect the species. One of the lesser-known protective elements provided by a herd is the strategy of muscle signaling.

Muscle signaling is the strategy adapted to counter a major flaw in the herd defense, that flaw being that all the best-tasting and easily killed young are gathered together by the herd for the benefit of the predator. He need not spend the energy to hunt for an easy kill.   They are already gathered together in one location and made available for him to eat.

The herd's muscle-signaling strategy counters the constant attacks on the needed members of the herd, especially the big cat's temptation to make the safest kill, the young and future of the species.   The strategy of the herd is to provide an alternative food source for the predator. A safer kill is offered, a kill that promises no risks of injury to the big cat.

This strategy uses the strength of thousands of sharp horns or kicking hoofs to divert the predator from attacking the young and the pregnant females. However, the herd knows that the lion must eat, so it provides an alternative source of food that will not fight back, and that alternative food source actually broadcasts a signal from its muscles directly to the hungry lion through muscle signaling.

Muscle signaling is an important survival tactic that was developed millions of years ago by herd animals to deal first with raptors and then with big cats. If the weak and the hurt and old signal the message "take me today, I will not fight" to the lion, and if they are taken and eaten, then the young of the species are safe for another day. That is another day for the young to grow and to get stronger. It is another day for the females to deliver a healthy new calf and for other females to be bred. The species lives by the weak sacrificing themselves for the good of their herd, their family, and their species.

This theory submits that sick, injured or weak herd animals are purposely signaling to the big cats that they are the safe, easy kill. This silent signaling by these animals is not voluntary; it is mandatory. Their reptilian brains demand that they be taken as the first source of food in its survival strategy for their herd. Humans, being a herd or tribe animal, send these same "take me today" distress signals out for the same reason that other herd animals do: for the survival of our children and our breeding females.

If you live in America or Europe and look out your window, your likelihood of seeing a big cat hunting for children and women is remote. If you live in the Western States and Canada, your chance of being killed is still remote if you are an adult male. However, if you are a child or a small female, your chances of being killed by a big cat sharply increases over that of a man. There are many big cats in mountainous areas that need to feed to survive. Most of the kills in these areas are what we expect: young children or small, fertile women that are not in the protection of the tribe. From about 1890 to date, about 40 small women and children have been known to be killed by the big cat that hunts in America: the cougar or mountain lion. These big cats weigh 90-160 lbs.

In the last five years, three children, ages 4 to 10, have been eaten by mountain lions in Texas, Colorado and Washington. Women, too, have been attacked and mauled recently.

Most of us have no fear that a big cat is going to eat a member of our family today.

You know this. You know it, but your ancient lower brain does not know it. It will never understand that you and your children are safe from the big cat.

Even if you tell yourself every day that you and your family are no longer part of that great migrating herd that is still being attacked by lions, your ancient brain will not listen to you. It is still on guard twenty-four hours a day to protect your family and the children that live near you by deploying its muscle-signaling defense strategy against your muscles. Your reptilian brain has never left the African savanna; it will never leave it. It will never cease in its desire to call the big cats to feast on you if you are weak, sick, depressed or stressed.

Chapter 6

Muscle Hierarchy

The "fight or flight" response of your body directly influences the placement of muscles on the lower brain's hierarchical list.

The muscle fibers within the striated (structural) muscles of your body have fast and slow twitch behaviors. The fast-twitch fibers contract with greater force and speed than do slow-twitch fibers; whereas, the slow-twitch fibers have greater endurance or stamina. Both types of fibers have some degree of flexibility, strength, power, endurance and the ability to grow and shrink in size. These five functions are needed to perform two muscle actions. The first is muscle contraction or flexion, and the second is muscle extension. They may perform these two actions alone or in supportive groupings. They perform these actions to give the body movement and direction. All striated muscle fibers provide body movements and direction with one goal: survival of your life force.

Your striated muscles are soldiers in the war for your survival. They only know a life of endless battles on your behalf. They live exclusively in the ancient brain's prehistoric world of fight, flight or death.

Fight Response of the Human Brain

Let us examine the ancient world of the striated muscle by looking at the body's fight response. Fight is more than kicking, hitting or attacking a threat or offensively protecting your family or your country. Fight is all positive life energy. It includes hunting, gathering, courting, mating, eating, playing, socializing, positioning yourself for recognition by peers and family, and working for needs and wants of yourself, your family, and your tribe. Fight is good.

The lower brain is willing to give loving attention and chemical inspiration to any muscle involved in the act of offensive survival (fight). The reptilian brain makes a partnership agreement with the muscles that rewards them for fighting for its forces. This is why it feels good to perform life-preserving activities, such as eating and socializing and helping your community (tribe).

The brain's chemical inspiration to the muscles can be observed when a 60-year-old grandmother lifts a car to rescue her grandson, or a rock climbing victim with a broken leg walks down a mountain to safety. The brain gives its attention to the muscles by supplying blood, nutrients and oxygen to its selected survival muscles. These are all part of the teamwork between the brain and the muscle in fight mode.

When the body is on the offensive, the brain gets positively involved because the lower ancient brain has an interest in the outcome of the fight that is larger than your self-preservation. Offense means all the lower brain's forces are winning, and the reptilian brain loves to win. When your brain and your muscles are in harmony, they are a winning team, a life-giving partnership where you benefit. "Partnership" is the word to remember if you want to be healthy and if you want to stay healthy over your lifetime.

Flight Response of the Human Brai ۱

Now let us examine the flight response of the reptilian brain and the structural muscles.

Flight or fleeing is more than running from an attacking animal or person. It includes cowering, avoidance of social responsibilities and conflicts, as in calling in sick when you're not, as well as all versions of saving face or saving one's self emotionally, including lying and the misrepresentations of your position in society. It even includes disengaging physically, as in laziness on the job or hiding in bed all weekend. Only when the brain rests, as in sleep or deep meditation, does the muscle rest within its partnership agreement with the lower brain. A muscle in flight mode, for any reason, has broken its life-giving partnership agreement with the lower brain.

Every muscle that is involved with flight runs a risk of being rejected by the lower brain. Flight is very bad for your body and mind. Just the dropping of your eyes so you will not make contact with another person is a major flight mode response to your reptilian brain. Whenever the flight response is activated, the positive partnership between the muscles and the brain are terminated, outright divorced. In the flight mode, the brain is at odds with your muscles. The reptilian brain then seeks to sacrifice one or more of your muscles on its hierarchal list.

All the healthy muscles of your body are constantly going into or out of the fight and flight response mode. A good night's rest would mean that most of the muscles upon rising are in the fight mode. One comes out of bed like a firefighter at the alarm, ready to win, ready for battle, ready to protect and defend the family and the tribe. The brain and body are in harmony. The partnership agreement between them is strong and vibrant.

Sadly, all one has to do is to be frightened by the morning news or hear some disheartening report, and every muscle that once was willing and able can change to the duck-and-cover flight mode. It does not have to be something apparent, like a verbal description of pending disaster over the television or radio, or a backhanded criticism of you from a loved one. A cold look from any tribe member can do it. This may be why research has shown that positive-thinking people are healthier than negative-thinking people. Positive thinkers can over-come flight mode activators, such as dirty looks or darting remarks, faster than negative people and thereby stay in the good fight mode for a longer time throughout the day and throughout the positive person's lifetime.

A fit and healthy muscle can handle short-term flight mode responses, but what must be avoided is long-term flight mode. Any time the reptilian brain perceives that a fight has turned against it, panic ensues, whether you are in a losing battle or you are asked to give an impromptu speech to justify your actions. Each time you go into the nega-tive "flight" mode, it is held in your muscle's memory.

Most people can look at someone and see the fight or flight response fixed in the muscle's memory. We can tell if a person is emotionally up (fight) or down (flight). What we are looking at that tells us this information is body language. Body language communi-cates either a fight mode or a flight mode. The body language that says a person is depressed shows muscles positioned for flight. Repetitive freezing of the muscles in flight mode causes long-term flight muscle memory, which then begins the process where the muscle broadcasts the "take me now, I will not fight" signal to the big cat telling it that your defenses are down and you will not fight for your life.

An example of flight mode response can best be demonstrated in a story of a young man who goes out alone into the jungle for the first time to hunt for a lion.   He is in fight mode. His tribe has given him encouragement, and he wants their respect and the respect of the single women when he returns with proof of his manhood, a lion.   He finds no lion the first day. As night falls, he climbs a tree for safety. As he sleeps, he has a dream that a deadly snake bites him. That morning he awakes shaken and worried. He searches the ground for snakes before he descends the tree.   Once on the ground and after a few hours of hunting, he finds lion tracks and he forgets about snakes. His eyes, ears and nose search the bush for lions. He spots a large male lion in the grass some 200 yards away. Sensing the young man, the lion charges him. Spear in hand, the young man holds his ground.   Every muscle in his body ripples with the positive energy that comes from the partnership agreement between the brain and its muscles   Then, in the grass, something moves, long and black. He loses concentration, his body jerks, and fear rushes in. He wants to run. He is now in full flight mode: panic.   His lowly reptilian mind races in panic. Run or Fight. He knows he cannot escape the lion or the snake. His lower brain must make a decision based on its perceived risk of death from each choice. If he believes he must return to fight mode to ensure his survival, he will fight. If he believes he should stay in flight mode, his brain will end its partnership with his muscles and they will not fight his battle but just flee in panic. As he is fleeing, the brain will plan its sacrifice of certain muscles to the lion. He may use his arms to shield himself or kick with a leg. Perhaps an arm or leg muscle may satisfy the lion's hunger.   The ancient brain uses the muscles first to fight, then for flight, and, finally, as a food-offering to a predator. Each time a person goes into flight mode, any muscle that has lost its relationship with the ancient brain becomes orphaned and is then prepared by the ancient brain to be sacrificed to the lion as the final defense strategy of the reptilian brain.

Dr. David Livingstone, (1813-1873) African missionary and explorer, who Henry

Stanley presumably found deep in the jungles of Africa, was lonely and chronically sick as he suffered from bouts with malaria. In 1844, the Doctor while helping a village protect their herds shot a lion that then turned and angrily attacked him. Livingstone wrote later about his experience, "(The lion) caused a sort of dreaminess (in me), in which there was no sense of pain, nor feeling of terror."

Livingstone did not try to fight the lion as it ripped into his flesh, he just gave up, as many sick herd animals do when they are attacked. He wrote of his thoughts of being locked in the jaws of a man-eating lion,
"I was wondering what part of me he would eat first." Livingstone's remarks about how peaceful he felt when being eaten may explain why so many herd animals, after having their muscle signaling answered by a big cat, just lay down and give up their life for the good of the herd once they are attacked.

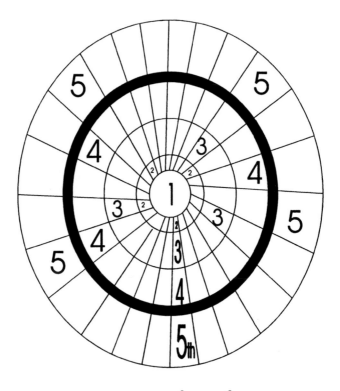

Rings of Life

Chapter 7

Morgan's "Rings of Life" Theory

The ancient herds of the African savanna were made up of many types of herd animals that had varying types of family structures. Some herds have one breeding bull and many cows; others had multiple breeding males. They all had one thing in common; they were always on the move to find new sources of food. As they traveled, the big cats preyed on them. As explained previously, herds developed a variety of defensive strategies. The most important strategy is the herd itself. The herd is a system of protective layers. Herds vary in their protective layers depending on the species within it. In some species this system was a basic layer of protection: the family layer, one bull and many females and young, or one breeding male and many non-breeding males, with their large horns, as the first defense; then the mothers, with their fast kicks, as the second layer; and then the calves, that can run, as the final defense.

Other herd animals, including humans, adopted a strategy of larger protective layers. These layers consist of five rings of defense. The first inner ring is the safest place to be in the herd. This is where the children are placed. We often hear the phrase, "Our children are our future." What this phrase is really saying is, "Our children are the future of our species and must be protected."

The second ring out from the center is the ring for nursing females, pregnant females and females that can become pregnant. These females protect their young from the big cat.

The third ring consists of non-breeding older females and older males. Its outer circumference includes breeding males that have fathered young and/or have grandchildren that are within the center ring and/or their mates who are within the second or third ring. In addition, in this ring are uncles and other males related by blood to the females and/or children. This ring protects the second and inner ring.

The fourth ring is where the strong, young, single males protect those in the first three rings. Human tribes place these young males in bands of warriors or in armies.

The riskiest place to be for muscle decline and pain is the fifth outer ring, where the sick, hurt, depressed, weak and outcasts can be found. The fifth ring ensures the species will survive from the daily attack of predators. These people in the fifth outer ring will be the first people to fall under attack and be sacrificed for the good of everyone (the whole tribe). People in this fifth ring have muscles that have given up the fight and are in full flight mode. They all are sending strong "take me" signals to attract hungry big cats.

How to Get Out of the Fifth Ring

It is very hard to move yourself out of the fifth ring. This is because you or at least your reptilian brain thinks you belong there. The only way to get yourself out of the ring is to petition the lower brain with Reflex-

Crafting. Reflex-Crafting has moved many people out of the fifth ring by addressing the lower brain with Sam Craft's techniques. You can use RC on yourself every day to get yourself out of the fifth ring. The lower brain has to believe that it made a mistake in order for you to get out of its grasp. Otherwise, you will need the daily help of others to persuade the lower brain to let you out.

Other people's positive energies must be given to you to tell the ancient brain that you, the person in the fifth ring, are needed by your family or your tribe for its survival. Being needed pulls you back towards the protective inner rings.

Negative energy by others has the opposite effect on your muscles. Human practices, such as name calling, racial labeling, rejecting, shunning, threats, gossiping and everyday put-downs, even in fun by a smiling friend or family member, tells the ancient brain that you, as a tribe member, are not needed in the inner rings but are sincerely wanted and needed in the outer fifth ring. Every human action, using positive or negative energy, works effectively over time to keep people within the inner rings or to push others to the outer fifth ring.

It may be that much of a person's daily thoughts and conversations are calculated by their reptilian brain to keep their family and friends within the safety of the inner rings and to protect their loved ones by pushing you and other tribe members out to the fifth ring. Gossiping about others is said to make up two-thirds of all adult conversation in America. Verbal attacks on others, because of their looks, dress, actions or beliefs, are a common topic of gossip. In fact, it is so common that it could be said that it is a natural human trait to daily push others to the outer fifth ring. Every day others are pushing you and sometimes you may feel the need to push yourself but once you are out there, you can wait a long time before you will find anyone willing to pull you back to safety.

Although you are being pushed by others on a daily basis, you are safely and firmly held in the inner rings when you are wanted and needed by your family or needed at work. You are given signals by those around you that your position within the four rings is necessary for your tribe's survival. These positive signals are picked up by the reptilian brain, and your muscles and tissues are rewarded by that brain. However, if you become sick or nonproductive or you come in conflict with your family or your tribe, you may be sent signals, either directly or subconsciously, by your family that you are not wanted or needed. You could be sent signals by your spouse or children that it would be better for everyone if you would go to the fifth ring. Even your doctor can send your brain this signal. Your muscles will then start, without your knowledge, calling to the lion.

Now, if you are wanted and needed and become sick, any member of your family and tribe can help you. They can come to you and pray or chant or hold you or lay hands on you and wish you well. This will keep you from moving to the fifth ring, or if you are in the fifth ring, they will move you towards the inner rings. While this positive signal from family or the tribe may not cure your illness, it does renew the life-giving partnership of your body to the reptilian brain and, thus, your brain gives your body everything that it needs so that, if it can, it will heal itself.

Today many hospitals are encouraging prayer and massage for the sick. It is well documented that patients recover faster and in some cases miraculously from these positive energies from family and tribe members.

To be and stay healthy, you must seek to keep yourself in line with positive energy forces. Depression, negative thinking, low self-esteem and flight muscle memory must be countered with positive energy signals to the lower brain. Reflex-Crafting and family and tribal acceptance counter negative forces. If a person wishes to escape being associated with the fifth ring, he or she needs to remain within the inner rings. To keep within the inner rings, you need to be a protector of children or the protector of a breeding female, or contribute to the tribe in such a way that you are rewarded by your tribe or your community or your family or at your work as a needed and wanted member. You must be told or signaled that you are needed and wanted in order to stay healthy.

If you do not get this positive energy from human sources or even from a pet, your reptilian brain will move you quietly and firmly to the outer fifth ring to be sacrificed. When you are there in the fifth ring, your reptilian brain will mesmerize your mind and fool you by giving you pleasure and the feeling that you are doing a wonderful thing by embracing the people and/or the culture of the fifth ring. This fifth ring mental state will cause you to purposely offend the people that love you so they will not help you. The more conflict you create within your family, the more secure and safe your lower brain makes you feel.

The fifth ring has a culture that the people in it conform to. It has norms of behavior. The culture of the fifth ring asks you to believe that sacrificing yourself for others is good and is your duty. You might hear your inner voice telling you to whine, preach at or criticize others, or you may lean on others or push your family members to the outer ring. You may be a caustic irritant to others but believe in your mind that you are helping them. You may have feelings that life is over or that life is not important and it is good just to give up. You might think about angels and how beautiful heaven is. You might look forward to reading the obituaries or feel that you need to visit the sick and/or work to help the dying or plan your funeral and buy a burial plot.

All seriousness aside, when you visit the lions at the zoo and you hear a little voice deep inside your head urging you to jump into their cage, it may be the time to do some Reflex-Crafting on yourself.

Recap

In review, your body was formed about 50,000 years ago by what your ancestors ate and what ate your ancestors. Your body form evolved as a plant eater and a herd member. You still are a plant eater and a herd member.

You have one large brain that has three functions. The upper brain, or rational brain, makes you human. It is the only brain with the powerful ability to learn or to copy the successful survival strategies of other life forms.

The mid-brain or mammalian brain system makes you want to care for children and family. It is the brain that plays and feels all emotions.

The oldest brain system is the reptilian brain. It uses four life forces for one grand purpose. That grand purpose is not to keep you alive but to keep your species alive. To do this, it uses one force to keep you alive, one force to keep your family alive, one force to keep your tribe alive and one overriding grand force to keep your species alive.

If you have an injury, a sickness or have a conflict with the overriding grand purpose to keep your species alive, you will be in conflict with your reptilian brain. This conflict of forces causes the reptilian brain to break its relationship with the muscles and tissues in your body. It has a hierarchal listing of all your muscles. Once one of your muscles is put on the bottom of this list, it begins the process of being sacrificed. In Reflex-Crafting, we believe that this is one source of muscle restriction and pain in your body. Reflex-Crafting your body will help you stay out of the fifth ring, and if you are in the fifth ring, it can help move you towards the inner rings.

The human brain needs and rewards people to go into the fifth ring. That is why there are so many people in it. Being pushed into the fifth ring is natural and at one time it was necessary for the survival of our species.

Chapter 8

Reflex-Crafting Muscle Theory

The Source of Muscle Pain

In ancient times, pain was thought to come from little devils with pitchforks who lived under the skin. Sneezing was thought to be an act of casting out these pain devils, the reason being the sicker a person was, the more sneezing they did. When a sick person sneezed, people would quickly say, "God bless you." This was said in the belief that it would keep the little pain devils from going back into its host's blessed body. Even today perfect strangers will say a blessing for you if you have sneezed. This positive act of being blessed, even by strangers, signals your lower brain that your tribe wants you.

Some believe that the organs of the body possess a consciousness. In or near one body organ in particular, the heart, some believe lives the True Mind. This True Mind finds peace within the clarity of unconditional love and rules over the brain and brings goodness to the brain that the eye cannot see. Some also believe that bad thoughts and illness are caused by bad experiences from past lives. These bad thoughts are caught and held in the conscious and unconscious mind. This is a new-age way of trying to explain why the body's muscles become sick and full of pain from no known cause or why bad things happen to good people. They believe that if a heart healer is focusing on the good energies of the body, then bad thoughts can be overcome and illness and/or pain can be cleansed from the body. What the healer is doing is telling the sick person that she is wanted and needed. Chanting, singing, drum beating, head patting and hugging are examples of positive energy being offered to the reptilian brain as proof that the person is wanted by the tribe in the inner rings and not needed in the fifth ring.

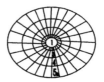

In Reflex-Crafting, we believe the instant a muscle is hurt, the normal healing process first begins with the injured person giving attention to a painful area by touching the area of pain or rubbing it. Then that person starts testing the muscle's flexibility, strength and movement. The muscle is then pampered for a certain amount of time to enable healing. When healed, it is back to a normal state and the person stops giving attention to that recovered healthy muscle.

Tri -Muscle Pain

There are three major conditions of muscles that we address with RC. They are the Normal Marked muscle, the Howler muscle and the Cloaked muscle. These tri-muscle conditions can occur in a muscle or within parts of a muscle. Using the charts in part two of this book, you can treat all these muscle conditions.

Normal Marked Muscles

In Reflex-Crafting, muscles that transmit their pain easily and directly from the site of the injury are called normal marked muscles. All healthy muscles indicate their pain directly to the brain and are marked by the brain as injured and in need of shielding. Examples of muscle marking are limping on a leg to shield the hurt hip, leg or foot. Covering, by placing one's hand over a hurt muscle, shields it from further injury. A mother kissing her hurt child is an act of covering, as is placing a Band Aid™ on an injury. Reflex-Crafting can sedate the pain in marked muscles and give a sense of calmness to the body.

Howler Muscles

The second muscle condition RC can address is called a howler muscle. This muscle sends out pain impulses, but the howler muscle is not hurt. These false pain impulses may be chronic. Howler muscle pain is a false pain signal. The pain is actually from another muscle that is not felt. Some injured muscles can cause otherwise healthy muscles to register pain to the brain. The howler muscle is marked by the brain as being in need of protection, but it is not hurt or sore. We have seen in our practice where a client may want his or her upper back massaged because of the pain that is perceived to originate from it, but that client suffered no back pain once the hip is Crafted. Some life-long muscle pain is, in fact, howler pain.

Howler pain can be briefly quieted by direct massage or visits to the chiropractor, but it will return to its painful state shortly after any treatment. No amount of direct massage, adjustments or surgery on the howler will stop it from falsely screaming.

Even when a person has had many years of muscle pain, Reflex-Crafting can, in seconds, locate the muscle that is actually causing the pain signal, and then, with a few treatments, quiet it and calm the howler muscle.

Cloaked Muscles

The third and the most dangerous muscle condition is called CMS, Cloaked Muscle Syndrome. With a cloaked muscle, there is little or no pain being signaled from the affected muscle. There may be pain involved and transmitted by howler muscles, but the cloaked muscle itself is usually silent. People that have cloaked muscle syndrome may report no problem or pain in the muscle.

When help is offered, they will earnestly ask that the person trying to help them to change the subject or not to touch the cloaked part of their body. Their request not to be helped is an indication of cloaked muscle syndrome.

A shielded, cloaked muscle is armored physically, mentally and emotionally. The reptilian brain even shields the muscle from the upper brain by blocking any soreness or pain from the rational upper brain. The cloaked muscle reports no pain when lightly touched, but the lower brain can supplant a fear of being touched, which is sent to the emotional brain and on to the upper brain. The CMS client uses every skill that his or her upper brain possesses to discourage getting help for the cloaked muscle. A client may go as far as verbally or physically instructing the body worker to work elsewhere in order to keep the cloaked muscle from being discovered. Sam Craft has been threatened and shown the door by more than a few of his clients that have CMS. People suffering with CMS have all three brains working together to keep their muscle cloaked. Many times the words that are used for shielding and protecting the cloaked muscle are enveloped in strong emotion. Depending on the personality of the client, the emotional brain may send feelings of aggression or even make outright threats against the person trying to help. For example, they may say: "I'm not paying you to mess with my shoulder, and I don't need a massage there," or deceptively distracting: "Can you move on to my feet now!" Its shielding may be cloaked in humor or defacing: "Don't bother there. In my family, we all have strong backs and weak minds." Aggressiveness, diversion, denial and humor are used by the brain to keep anyone from releasing the armored, cloaked muscles.

Muscle cloaking is an abnormal aftermath to the normal process of healing. There are three progressive stages that a muscle passes through to become fully cloaked. The first stage is "muscle shielding."

This stage begins with a person physically protecting the muscle for some time beyond its need for protection. A person may place their hand on the muscle while talking or when they feel insecure or tired. They may wear a coat or other protective clothing, and on a hot day may refuse to wear lighter clothing because it does not offer them enough shielding protection. They may walk with an unnecessary cane or other device to shield the muscle from use. Shielding can present itself both physically and/or emotionally. Muscle shielding is a reptilian brain function. In most cases, the upper thinking brain does not realize that it is occurring.

If shielding occurs over a long period of time, the protected muscle enters the second stage called "mummification." These muscles are so protected that they stop being used for movement and motion. They are being mummified, while still alive, by the reptilian brain, wrapped in layers of hardening fascia and filled with the sharp and sometimes pain-causing crystals and other embalmment and petrifying agents. A mummified muscle begins to be actively shielded by the full powers of the upper rational brain as it is being sacrificed by the lower reptilian brain.

People with a mummified muscle will shield that muscle by making clever and rational excuses for not using that muscle or for not getting help to recover the movement in the muscle. They make and then break appointments to get help. You might hear excuses based on age, like: It's just old age setting in. Excuses based on work, like: I'm too busy to get a massage. Excuses like: My back is as strong as an ox, you should feel how hard it is!

At some point a mummified muscle can be very painful but the joining of the forces of both the upper and lower brains against the muscle to keep it from returning to a healthy condition is hard for the victim to overcome. Sufferers just live with it, they take pills and complain. If they are told that they can get relief, they hesitate to get help or scoff at the treatment.

The third stage of the cloaking of the muscles is the "zombie stage," the living dead. Muscle cloaking is defined in Reflex-Crafting as the process in which a muscle is prepared by the brain to be sacrificed. We see this mostly in the elderly where they shuffle their feet and bend over while walking. We also see it in those of middle age in the smaller muscles of their shoulders, neck and spine. This stage is noted by the person changing his or her posture or body movement to compensate for the loss of use of the muscles. Some will change their entire lifestyle. Most will deny that they have a problem or need help.

Mentally the person may refuse to recognize that the muscle's motion and flexibility ever existed. They avoid touching the muscle, and when asked why they sit, stand, walk, or bend in such an odd way, they say that they have always done it that way. After this point, CMS is at full onset and many muscle problems that were hidden become known. People fall down. They cannot open a can with a can opener. They cannot turn their head while driving. They can't walk without dragging their feet. Sometimes a friend or family member points out the problem and tells them to do something about it, only to be rebuffed or ignored. With full CMS, all three brains work together in their effort to cloak the muscle and keep it cloaked.

The emotional brain may scream with anger at anyone trying to help the victim. If forced to, the cloaked person reluctantly makes an appointment with a doctor or chiropractor, and, if they are lucky, a Reflex-Crafter, to get help.

A chiropractor will adjust their spine. The doctor may tell them to exercise, take pills or will refer them to a physical therapist or chiropractor for manipulation. What does the RC master or the reader of this book do?

Knowing why the muscles have cloaked, you can proceed to communicate with the three controlling forces that keep the muscle cloaked, the three forces that you will work with: your rational mind, your reptilian mind, and the involved muscles. Each force must be overcome in order to relieve cloaked muscle syndrome. The upper brain can be persuaded to seek help, but the mid-brain and reptilian brain want absolutely no help.

When working on yourself or others, to be successful the rational thinking brain must first be convinced that CMS is not a normal condition of aging; secondly, that CMS can be treated and reversed and finally that the upper brain can see the logic in treating the hands and feet before working on any problem area on the body.

These three steps are accomplished by talking to the upper brain and presenting evidence, such as this book and retelling other people's testimonies. The hardest part of getting the upper brain to switch sides is to convince it that the pain that the person feels in their hands and feet that is associated with Reflex-Crafting is necessary for its own good. You must start with positive communications to the rational upper brain and use rational thinking to ease the fight-or-flight conflict of the mind by persuading the rational thinking mind that there is nothing to fear or fight when the hands and feet are treated and the pain hits the brain. This seems odd at first thought, but to deal with the irrational reptilian mind, the rational mind must take over the driver's seat of the brain. It must take control of the reptilian brain.

Next, the reptilian brain must be addressed. If the muscles are cloaked, then the reptilian brain and body are at odds with one another. This is a fight for survival. The lower brain believes that the muscles should stay cloaked and should be sacrificed. In animals, we know of some species of lizards that drop off their tails as a sacrificial muscle decoy. In the lowly lizard's reptilian brain-to-body hierarchal structure, when being scared or in danger, the reptilian's brain will sacrifice and drop one-third of its body. Every muscle in its tail is sacrificed to appease the predator. Then the disembodied muscles in the tail twist and turn so that they distract any predator from the fleeing lizard.

There are examples of mammals that sacrifice muscle and tissue, such as wolves, foxes and wildcats, that will chew off a foot or leg to escape the grip of an iron trap, further amplifying the reptilian's brain vs. body struggle for survival.

Start communicating with the reptilian brain by using the charts in this book to find the RC points for the muscle that is cloaked. You can identify cloaked muscles by searching the hands and feet for these RC points that relate to patterns of pain. Using the four Reflex-Crafting techniques in a step-by-step process will address the fight-or-flight subconscious fears of the ancient brain. And the techniques will work to reassign the cloaked muscle to a new position on the hierarchy list.

When it comes to the hierarchy of human muscles, we have some clues as to what happens when fear or stress occurs. We know any time a Reflex-Crafter touches an area on the body and brings relief to that area or to another part of the body by sedating an RC point, it progressively builds a sense of trust to the total brain, letting the thinking, rational brain know, by receiving pain, that relief will be felt. With each success, the ancient brain becomes more accepting to touch; thus, the lower brain moves into an open, relaxed state and releases the cloaked muscle from its place on the hierarchy list. Reflex-Crafting techniques work more effectively on pain over time, as the muscle is moved up in rank on the list.

Why?

It must be made clear that once a muscle begins the cloaking process, your reptilian brain does not want your muscle to ever heal or for you to feel better. Never. Your very own brain battles you to keep you sick. It wants to put more muscles on its list, not less. It wants to use you so that it can protect your children, your family and your tribe from harm. It pushes you and manipulates you so it can protect the ones that you love by sacrificing you. It believes that the lions are outside your door and they must be fed.

You are on a one-way trip to the outer fifth ring. The reptilian brain will do whatever it can, even lie to you to keep you on this path. The brain will make you lie about your pain and make you deny to anyone that is trying to help you that you have a problem. All this is rational and justified to the irrational ancient reptilian brain.

The Rings of Life and the four forces of the reptilian brain applies to more than just muscle sacrifice. We see these same compulsions to move to the fifth ring in people with depression, addictions and those that have suffered the loss of a child or spouse. We see it from time to time in those that have lost their job or who have retired. High stress, conflict, emotional eating and any injury to the body can stimulate the ancient brain to push you to the outer ring. This is a normal and effective way to protect others in your family. When you are hurting and feel unwanted, your reptilian brain can treat you as if you are its sacrificial tail.

How to Uncloak

The worry and fear that we foresee happening to us tomorrow, combined with everything that actually happened to us yesterday, remains within us. It remains in our muscles. This retained injury can occur from emotional conflicts with life, such as when we have a conflict with our spouse, family or with our community. Furthermore, a muscle can be cloaked if it falls from its place on the hierarchal list because of under-use. Either way, the stress must be unlocked from our muscle's memory if we are to undo the damage that it has caused. The Reflex-Crafting points, referred to as RC points in this book, are located in our hands and feet. They hold these memories long after the injury-retaining cloaked muscle has armored itself and the reptilian brain has moved the muscle on to its sacrificial hierarchal list.

When a Reflex-Crafter contacts an RC point on the hand or foot, that point signals the brain with a jolt of pain. By rubbing and activating the RC points on the hand and foot, we directly interface with the marked muscles and with cloaked muscles in the legs, neck, arms and torso of the body. Both the marked and the cloaked muscle will transfer its pain to the point on the hand that is being activated. If the pain in the muscle is intense, then the pain at the RC point will be equally or more intense. After activation of the RC points, the affected muscle opens a channel of communication with the reptilian brain. Reflex-Crafting communicates to the lower brain that the cloaked muscle is needed by the body and at the same time sends a message that the person is needed and wanted by the tribe. It awakens the upper brain to the fact that the muscle is cloaked. Sedative pressure is then placed on the RC point, which relaxes the muscle, and the pain subsides.

When a cloaked muscle drops its

armor, all three brains release their hold on it. Cloaked muscles can be directly addressed by Reflex-Crafting to release all emotional bindings and any referred pain that has been sent to a howler muscle. Both muscles are then pain-free. After a few treatments to remove the mummy wrappings, all cloaking is reversed and a new partnership with that muscle is formed with the reptilian brain. This partnership moves the muscle to a higher, healthier position on the reptilian brain's hierarchy list.

Understanding RC Pain Points

Reflected sunlight in a mirror originates from the sun, not from a point inside the mirror. Nevertheless, the glare is just as painful to the eyes. Pain points, called RC reflex points in the hands or feet, mirror any muscle pain that originated in the body's structural muscles. If there is no injury or disease in the hands or feet that is causing pain, then the pain in these RC points is reflected pain. The original source of these pain points in the hands and feet is from marked muscles or cloaked muscles elsewhere in the body.

You need to know that all RC pain points in the hands and feet are known as reflected or ghost pain. That is to say, it is not real pain; the pain that is felt does not exist in the feet or hands. This cannot be overstated, so I will repeat it: There is nothing that hurts in the feet or hands. There is no real pain whatsoever in the hands or feet, as there is no real sun inside the mirror. The light in the mirror is only the reflection of the real sun.

Once the sun goes down, the mirror goes dark. Once the pain leaves the muscle, the pain leaves the foot or hand. The reason I repeated myself is that the pain is just as real in the mind of a person as true nerve-induced pain. RC pain has been said to feel like fire, pins and needles and, at times, causes painful itching. Because it is concentrated in RC points, this reflected pain can and does hurt as much as if it were real pain originating from the hand or foot.

A muscle that is eleven inches long and fully cloaked and armor-protected can transfer all of its pain to the hand or foot in a point that is the size of a dime. A muscle that is full of pain is able to concentrate that pain in an inch of flesh. Hitting that painful spot on the foot may cause a person to lift off the massage table due to the pain. After working the RC points on the hand or foot, the pain-causing muscle will uncloak, and then that uncloaked muscle can produce as much pain as the RC point. This may cause the client to believe that the Reflex-Crafter has caused the pain, but, in fact, the Reflex-Crafter has just uncloaked it. This muscle can now be manipulated by further Reflex-Crafting techniques to reprogram its memory to a pain-lessening state.

Once the pain is relieved, it is normal for people to say that they have a new pain in another location of their body. If this new pain is relieved, then another pain may be noticed on the body, and then another after that one is released. Luckily, Reflex-Crafting can be used on a daily basis because it is so simple to use. Generally, everyone can be calmed by the sedation technique to build the bond of trust with the lower brain and to make the next treatments more effective.

In reviewing what has been covered, muscle cloaking, as defined in RC, is when the muscle is in the ultra-slow process of self-atrophy. These muscles are being mummi-fied while alive. A cloaked muscle is on the bottom of the reptilian brain's hierarchy list, and, by being so, is being readied for lion food by the reptilian brain.

Reflex-Crafting, when used on the hands or feet, brings relief to a low-priority muscle. It progressively builds up the priority of that muscle on the reptilian brain's muscle hierarchical list. With each success, the brain becomes more accepting of these orphaned muscles, causing Reflex-Crafting techniques to become more effective over time in renewing muscles and stopping any associated pain. The person feels well and happy as the partnership between the brain and the muscles is once again instated.

Again, we are stating that all healthy muscles hurt or become sore when worked hard. Because a muscle was hurt or is sore does not mean that it is going to cloak. Cloaking is part of the survival process of the ancient brain. Only it knows what, if any, muscles it will cloak. The good news is that common sore and stiff muscles can be treated with Reflex-Crafting to relax and return them to their normal state and that most cases of CMS can be treated and reversed by Reflex-Crafting by using its simple techniques to communicate with the reptilian lower brain.

Reflex-Crafting
Part Two

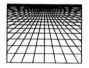

RC Guideline

When you are applying sedative pressure
to a point on your foot, hand or body and
you feel the muscle under your thumb or finger
kick or hit back at you, that muscle is cloaked or
is trying to cloak.

Give special attention to that muscle.
Have a loved one tell you that you are needed
and wanted by your family as you work that area.

Work that RC Point or RC Grid square often.

The Four Techniques for the Crafting of Reflex Points

There are only four simply applied techniques to learn in Reflex-Crafting. They were chosen by Sam Craft to be used in the Reflex-Crafting of the body and its RC pain points. Each technique uses light to heavy pressure to push into the tissues of the body.

There are two active techniques. They are used by working a tight circle on an area of the hands and feet under the tips or pads of the thumbs or fingers. The first Active Technique is called Active RC Crushing.

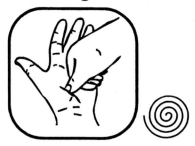

Active RC Crushing

The next Active Technique is called Active RC Pinching.

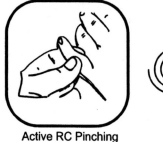

Active RC Pinching

The next two RC techniques are **Sedative.** They do not use rotation but instead use the thumb and finger to pinch down or press down on the hands and feet and body.

Sedative RC Crushing is used on the whole body.

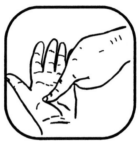

Sedative RC Crushing

Sedative RC Pinching is used on the parts of the body that can be squeezed between the thumb and fingers.

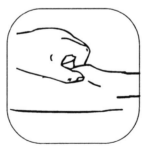

Sedative RC Pinching

Chapter 9

Reflex Crafting Techniques & Charts

Using Reflex-Crafting techniques on yourself, you can do the following:

1) Discover weaknesses in your structural muscles
2) Provide a quick, systematic approach to calming your body and mind
3) Reclaim muscle tone and performance (uncloak)
4) Stop pain, both chronic (reoccurring) and acute (new)
5) Start the process of moving out of the fifth ring.

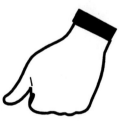

By using Reflex-Crafting pain-relief techniques, the brain manufactures endorphins, which are natural pain-killers that block nerve reception, thereby relieving your pain. The brain is additionally addressed to relax the muscle and readjust the muscle's position. Frequent applications with light pressure will give you better results than if you use one heavy application that could cause you or others a great deal of discomfort. If your muscles are painfully tender, you should start your Reflex-Crafting session with the first technique that sedates the sore muscle. This is called **Sedative RC Crushing**.

When using **Sedative RC Crushing,** You use either one or more fingers and the thumb, or just a finger or thumb, to apply steady pressure to the RC points and tissues on the hands, feet and body. There is no circling or lateral movement.

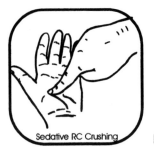

Sedative RC Crushing   Fig. 1

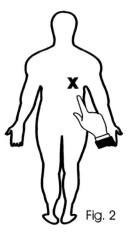

Fig. 2

Begin your RC session by pressing your finger on a painful spot on your body to mark it (fig.2). Then refer to the charts located at the end of this chapter. The charts are comprised of three parts that show the RC paths for the muscles of the neck/torso, arms and legs.

As an example, if you find a painful spot in your lower back, check the neck and torso charts to see what muscles are near your sore spot. If you find a painful spot in the arms, check the arms charts. If you find a painful spot on the legs, check the leg charts. You may need to check the leg and the torso charts if the pain involves muscles covered in both areas.

The charts in each section will show the

position of the reflex points (RC points) as a black band over the release area. An example would be the neck/torso chart. It will show a black band over the reflex points that correspond with a muscle on the neck or the torso.

The charts (fig.3) show both the feet and the hands. For maximum benefit, you should work the RC points on the same side as the pain is in your body.

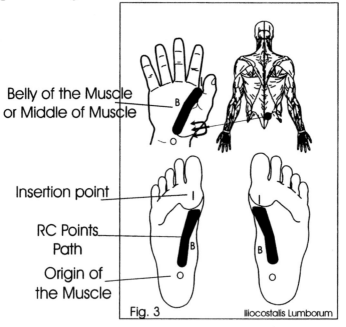

Belly of the Muscle or Middle of Muscle

Insertion point

RC Points Path

Origin of the Muscle

Fig. 3

Iliocostalis Lumborum

To work the paths, simply press into any point along the selected black path until you feel pain (fig.4). If you do not feel pain, release the pressure and move down the path. Then, using your thumb, press into the flesh. Hold firm, even pressure for at least 15 seconds, but preferably until the pain releases either in the spot that you're pressing on or the muscle relaxes that you're trying to release. Then release the pressure. Move down the black pathway using this technique on each RC pain point that you find.

To reduce uncomfortable feeling of pain, take deep breaths and let them out slowly. After a couple deep breaths, the pain diminishes and is tolerable.

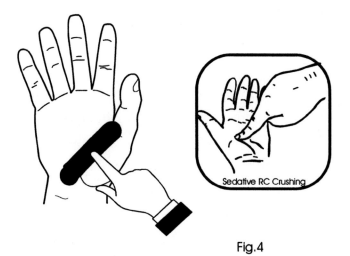

Sedative RC Crushing

Fig.4

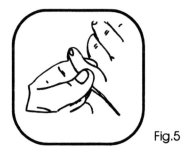

Fig.5

Another technique that can be used is **Active RC Pinching** (fig.5). **Active RC Pinching** is used on areas of the hands or feet that can be pinched, like between the fingers and toes and along the wrists. When using this crab-like grip, pinch the area you're trying to address, whether it is the tissue between your fingers or just your finger. Grab it. **Active RC Pinching** is never used on the body itself.

After locating a painful area, grab the tissue and roll it between your fingers for 15 seconds. Then move to another area, following the designated area on the charts, and repeat the technique. Try to grind the tissue between your fingers as if you were trying to break a piece of chalk into powder. When pressing in with your finger or your thumb, roll in a small, tight circle, not in a large circle. Then move along the path, repeating the technique.

The next technique is **Sedative RC Pinching,** which is identical to **Active RC Pinching,** except there is no circling movement. Steady pressure is used.

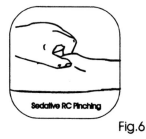

Sedative RC Pinching

Fig.6

The fourth technique is called **Active RC Crushing** (fig.7). In this technique, the thumb or the finger is pressed into the flesh on an RC point on the charted path. When using the thumb or finger, small circles are made where you are pressing while applying pressure for 15 to 20 seconds. Then lift and move down the path.

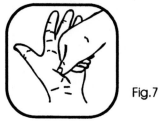

Fig.7

107

We do not use thumb-walking in Reflex-Crafting. Thumb-walking is defined as using the thumb to travel over the flesh on the path without being lifted out of the flesh. With **Active RC Crushing** (fig.8), we lift the thumb up from the flesh and then reapply pressure.

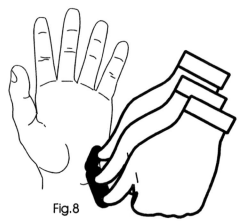

Fig.8

When doing the Active technique always press in deep and circle with the tips of the thumb or fingers. Never rub the skin,as rubbing could cause a blister on the skin.

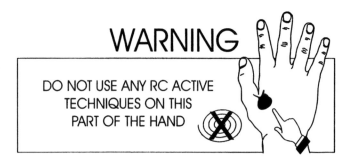

WARNING

DO NOT USE ANY RC ACTIVE TECHNIQUES ON THIS PART OF THE HAND

Reflex-Crafting Sciatica Pain:

To address sciatica pain that involves the hip, all four of the pain relief techniques will be used. The **Active RC Crushing/Active RC Pinching** methods should be done for at least 15 seconds at each point along the path. For the sedation techniques, **Sedative RC Crushing/ Sedative RC Pinching**, you will hold the point until your pain subsides.

After completing each pain relief method, stand up and move around to see if your pain has diminished. This will help you identify which pain relief techniques are most effective for you, Active or Sedative. Expect some immediate relief from pain, better movement and more flexion in the involved muscles.

When you are working on your sore

muscles of the hip, have someone else do the sedative pain relief techniqu? for you using only the Sedation methods.

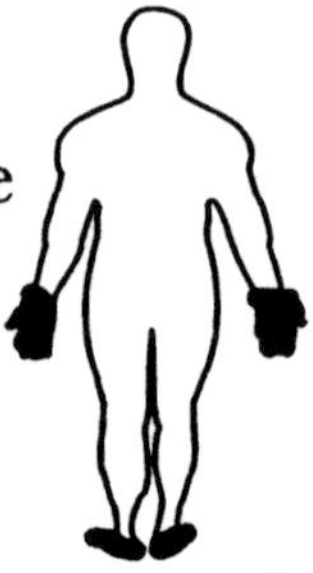

In Reflex-Crafting, we do not use the **Active RC Crushing** or **Active RC Pinching** anywhere but on the feet and most parts of the hands (fig 9).

Fig.9

The following is how to stop sciatica involving the left hip by working on RC points on the left hand. The first point you are going to work on is the big joint on the left thumb where it joins the hand. We're going to work 360 degrees around the thumb's large joint.

Begin by using the **Active RC**

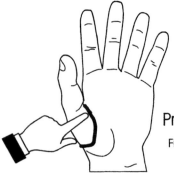

Press on the bone

Fig.10

Crushing Technique to work completely around the joint. You will be searching for sore spots. Once you've worked completely around the joint, use the Sedation techniques over this same path.

Remember, the Active technique is using the tip and/or pad of your finger or thumb and circling for 15 seconds, moving and finding a new point, and continuing in 15-second treatments around the thumb joint. The Sedation technique is simply pressing in and holding until the pain subsides--usually this takes 15 or 20 seconds--then moving along the path. Press and hold again until you come completely around the thumb.

Remember to work completely around the joint, including on the web between the joint and the first finger. Then use a Sedation technique on each point that you used the Active technique on until the pain subsides.

Next, work on the wrist itself, palm side up. Working on this point, we use the **Active RC Pinching** Technique on the little finger side of the wrist, starting at the wrist, to about halfway into the wrist and two inches down. Press and circle for 15 seconds, then release. Work this area using the **Active RC Pinching** technique over the black path.

Using the **Active Pinching** technique, you can work all the way from the base of the hand up to the base of the little finger.

The last technique is **Sedative RC Pinching**. By grabbing the tissue between the thumb and your first finger, we will sedate the muscles of the hip. We hold this point until the pain subsides.

Next, we sedate down the thumb side of the hand. (Fig. 11)

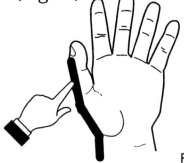

Fig. 11

112

Grab firmly, holding to the sides. Do this over the entire length of the side of the hand until you reach just above the wrist, and holding until the pain subsides, and then release.

--ooOoo--

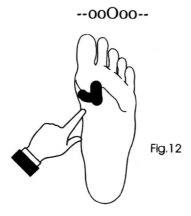

Fig. 12

To address the RC points in the foot, we will now go to your left foot. (fig.12). Using the charts, locate the muscle path on the chart. You can begin by pressing on any RC points on the foot that corresponds to the points on the chart. You will use the **Active RC Crushing** Technique.

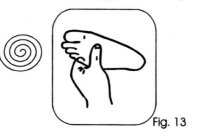

Fig. 13

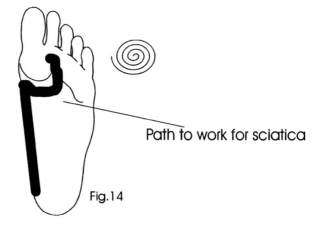

Path to work for sciatica

Fig.14

For sciatica, you want to press into the muscle path right in between the large toe joint at the ball of the foot, to the end of the ball of the foot, towards the instep. You will need to press against the bone and push in deep. This should feel uncomfortable when you're pressing there if you have sciatica. Press hard, making small circles with your thumb. Then stop, lift your thumb and move to the next point on the path.

As you did with the joint in the hand, you will work 360 degrees around the ball of the foot. If you find lumps here, continue to work on those lumps. Press and circle, lift, press and circle around until the pain diminishes. Continue to do this all the way around the joint.

Once you have covered the whole 360-degree joint area completely, you need to retrace your path by simply pressing into the flesh using the **Sedative RC Crushing** Technique and cover the same points again. This will sedate the muscles of the hip.(fig. 15)

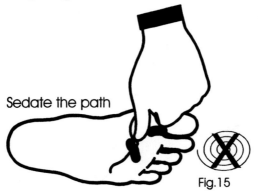

Sedate the path

Fig.15

Next, to stop sciatic and hip pain, you will work on the sole of the foot. You will start with the pad of the ball joint. Use the **Active RC Crushing** Technique and work the whole pad, including in and under and between the bone. This is like the large joint of the thumb. You work it doing the Active Technique. Keep working and hold firmly for about 20 seconds on each point, then move to a new point and actively pinch it. We continue doing this until we've covered virtually every square inch of path around the ball of the foot.

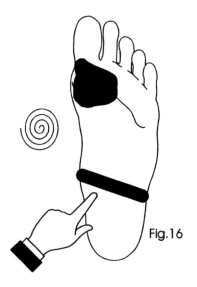

Fig.16

Now you are going to shift and move down to where the bottom of the foot is the narrowest,(fig.16) from the center of your foot over to the points on the path for the hip. You simply massage this firmly using the **Active RC Crushing** Technique. Then move to a new point, massage 15 seconds, and then continue to a new point.

116

Once you have covered all these points with the Active Technique, we simply go back and use the **Sedative RC Crushing** Technique over the same area. Hold each point steadily for 20 seconds until the pain subsides. Move to a new point, press and hold for 20 seconds until the pain subsides.

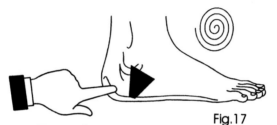

Fig.17

To release the hip, go to the reflex points located close to the heel (fig.17). Locate these points on the back of the heel and on the side of the foot. Start by pressing into the side of the heel, making circles, using the **Active RC Crushing** Technique. Crush each RC point for 15 seconds. Still on the side of the foot, press against the bone firmly for 15 seconds. Continue doing this to cover every square inch, including the tendon. You will want to get your finger right on the tendon and actively pinch it. Press against the tendon sideways. This is the Achilles tendon. Press in deep. Rub the tissue beneath the skin. Find a new spot; do the same thing. Find a new RC point; do the same thing, repeating for 15 seconds each time.

Now come back and address the same Reflex-Crafting points you just covered by doing the passive **Sedative RC Crushing** Technique. Press in firmly and hold till the pain diminishes greatly. Move to the next point and press in and hold 15 seconds or at least until the pain diminishes greatly. Press in and hold. The pain should be much, much less at this point.

After the Reflex-Crafting points on both the left foot and left hand are released, it is time to release the left hip.

Hip Releasing Techniques on the Body

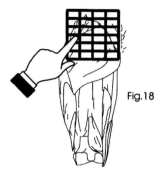

Fig. 18

To release the hip, (fig. 18) you need to imagine a grid of small, finger-sized squares on the hip area. Using only the two passive Sedation Techniques, you can start just about anywhere on the hip that is sore. You press in firmly. If you find no discomfort in that square, you move to another square looking for an area that hurts. Assuming that this square is painful, you will hold the pressure point at least 20 seconds or until the pain starts to subside. Then you simply move to the next square and press. You are starting to form a pain grid. That way, you can check every square inch of the buttocks and the hip without missing an RC pain point. If there's no pain, move on to the next square. If there is pain there, hold until the pain subsides; then find a new sore square on your grid.

Press in, hold till the pain diminishes, and then move on until all squares of the grid have been tested and released.

After you have made a pain grid by pressing on the hip, take your finger and press laterally into the hip socket itself. Generally, when you press here you will feel some referred pain or discomfort in the middle of the low back. Don't be alarmed. This is natural. If this point is very painful, hold it until the pain lessens. Then check around the area to see if there is another sore spot in that area. If there is, then press and hold until the pain diminishes.

That concludes Reflex-Crafting of the left hip. To do the right hip, just repeat the techniques on the right hand, foot and hip.

Recap:

Remember, when using the **RC Active Crushing** or the **RC Active Pinching Techniques**, do them for at least 15 to 20 seconds.

When using the **RC Sedative Crushing** or **RC Sedative Pinching** method, hold a steady pressure until the pain subsides.

By following these four pain-relief techniques, you can expect some immediate relief from pain, better movement and flexibility.

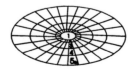

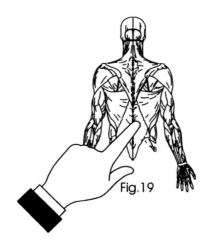

Fig.19

Reflex-Crafting the Lower Back

All four of the pain relief techniques will be used to relieve pain in the lower back. Again, the **Active RC Crushing** method should be done for at least 15 to 20 seconds at each point. And for the Sedation techniques, hold the point until the pain subsides.

After completing each pain relief method, stand up and move around to see if your pain has diminished. This will help you to identify which pain relief techniques are most effective for you.

To work on your lower back, have someone else do the pain-relief techniques on the grid for you. Use only the Sedation methods, never **Active RC Crushing**. If the pain does not diminish when pressing on a specific area, do not continue. Check with your doctor.

Releasing Back Pain through the Hand

You will start where the thumb joins the hand at the big knuckle. What we want to do is do the active technique on this knuckle just like we did on the hip, and we can start by addressing the knuckle between the thumb and the first finger. We're using the **Active Crushing** technique. You work completely around the thumb 360 degrees.

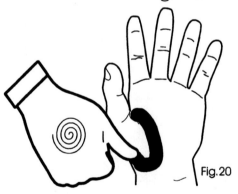

Fig.20

Referring to Figure 20, next you will work the area on the palm where the thumb joins the hand and the thumb starts. On the left hand, press right off the bone so that you press into the tissue just below the pad of the thumb. Use the **Active RC Crushing** Technique first for about 15 seconds. Then stop.

Now press in and use the Sedation Technique for at least 15 seconds or until the pain diminishes, and then move towards the index finger. Press in again, rotate 15 seconds, release, press in, hold till the pain greatly diminishes. You repeat this process along the path until you reach the finger.

Moving to the wrist, you want to work a grid pattern that entails half the wrist and half the palm on the thumb side of the hand.(fig 21). Use the **Active RC Crushing** technique to press each square in this grid. This grid area on the wrist and hand affects the lower back. **Sedative RC Crush** each square for 15 seconds, whether or not there's any pain in each square.

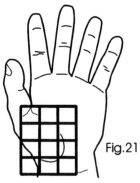

Fig.21

Now re-covering the same area, locate painful points where you will use the **Sedative** technique. Hold these points until the pain is almost gone. Then move to the next grid square, press and hold until the pain is almost gone. Repeat by moving to the next grid square, press in and hold until the pain greatly diminishes. Do this along the black path as shown on the chart in Chapter 9.

--ooOoo--

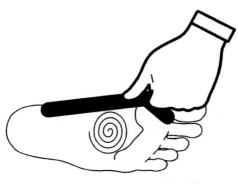

Fig.22

Reflex-Crafting the Foot for Back Pain

Next, we move to the RC points on the foot.(fig.22) Using the whole area of the arch on the bottom of the foot, you're going to start in between the big toe and the ball of the foot. Pressing against the top of the ball joint, use the Active Crushing Technique for 15 seconds. Moving down from the toe towards the heel, actively crush each point along the way for 15 seconds.

After the path has been actively crushed, it needs to be sedated. Sedate the path that you have previously crushed by holding each point until the pain diminishes greatly, moving to the next point to repeat the technique for 15 seconds each.

Once both the hand and foot have been addressed, move to the area of the back that is sore and make your imaginary grid over the sore spot (fig.23). Use the **Sedative RC Crushing** Technique to sedate each square in the grid. If you do not have someone to help you do this, you can lean against a table corner, lie on a golf ball or use a broom handle to hold for 15 to 20 seconds on each square.

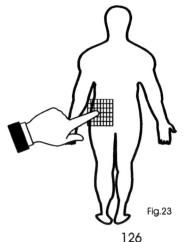

Fig.23

You Have Three Minds
That Care for You.
To Find Peace and Happiness
You Must
Meet Each of Their Needs.

Reflex-Crafting Charts
For the Neck, Torso, Arm and Leg

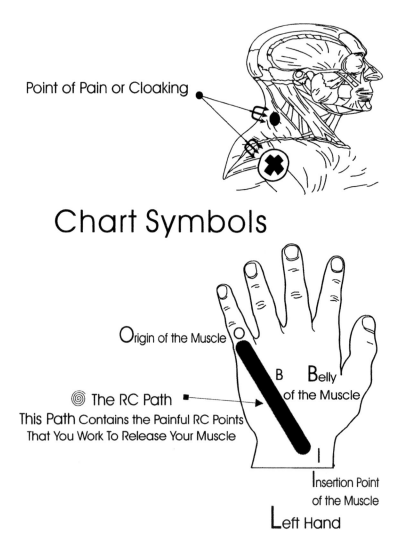

Point of Pain or Cloaking

Chart Symbols

Origin of the Muscle

B   Belly
of the Muscle

The RC Path
This Path Contains the Painful RC Points
That You Work To Release Your Muscle

I
Insertion Point
of the Muscle

Left Hand

Reflex-Crafting the Neck

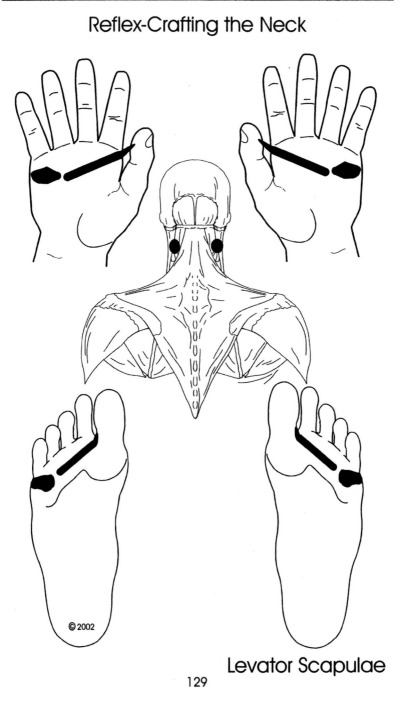

© 2002

Levator Scapulae

Reflex-Crafting the Neck

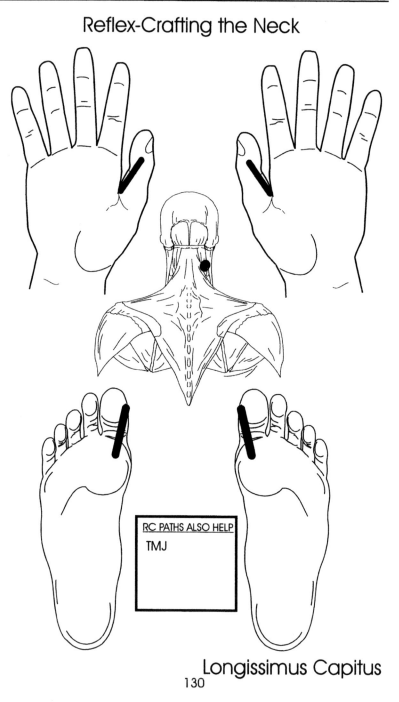

RC PATHS ALSO HELP

TMJ

Longissimus Capitus

Reflex-Crafting the Neck

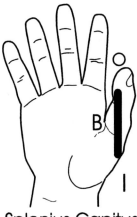

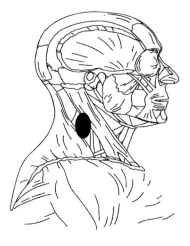

Splenius Capitus

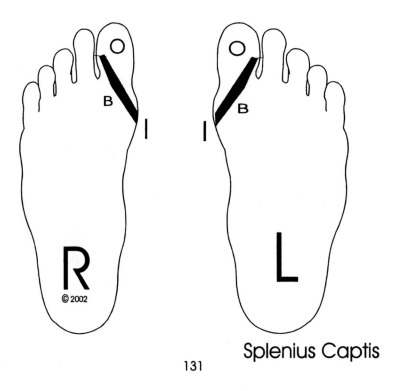

Splenius Captis

Reflex-Crafting the Neck

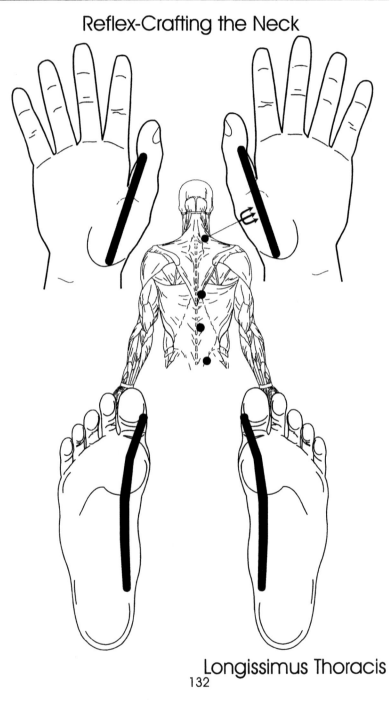

Longissimus Thoracis

Reflex-Crafting the Neck

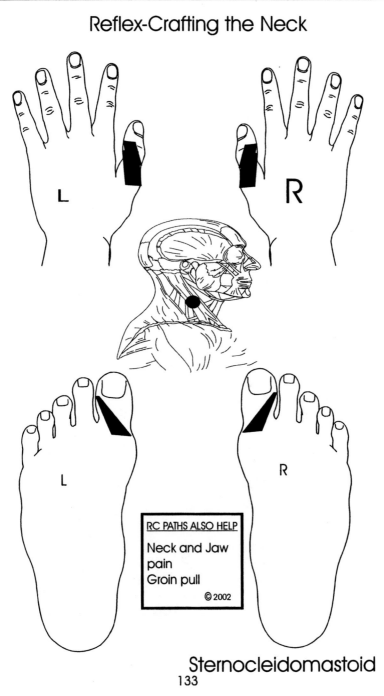

RC PATHS ALSO HELP

Neck and Jaw
pain
Groin pull

© 2002

Sternocleidomastoid

133

Reflex-Crafting the Neck and Torso

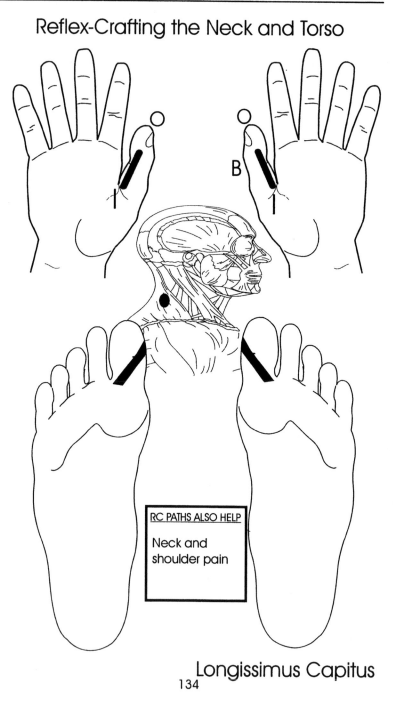

B

RC PATHS ALSO HELP

Neck and
shoulder pain

Longissimus Capitus

Reflex-Crafting the Neck and Torso

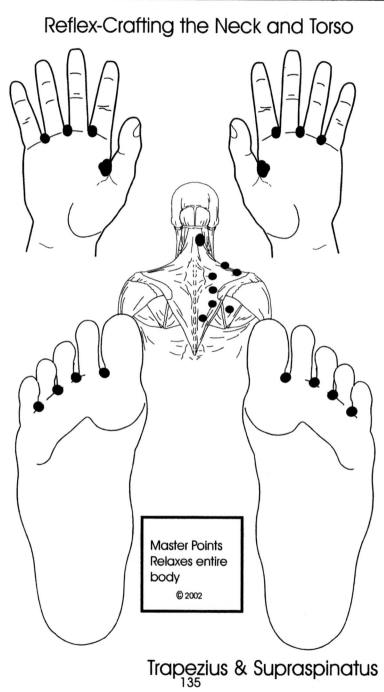

Master Points
Relaxes entire
body

© 2002

Trapezius & Supraspinatus

Reflex-Crafting the Back

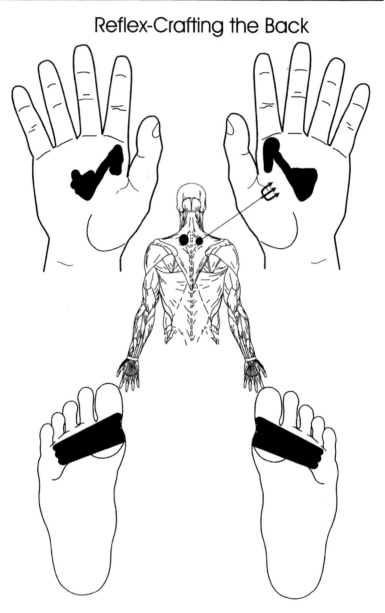

Muscle of the Back

Rhomboidus

Reflex-Crafting the Back

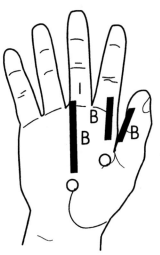

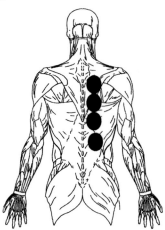

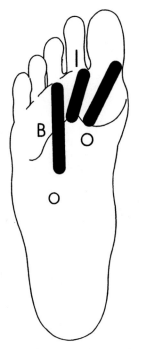

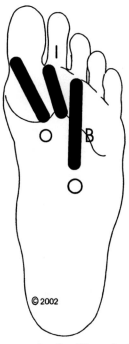

© 2002

Muscle extends Vetebral Column   **Iliocostalis Thoricis**

Reflex-Crafting the Back

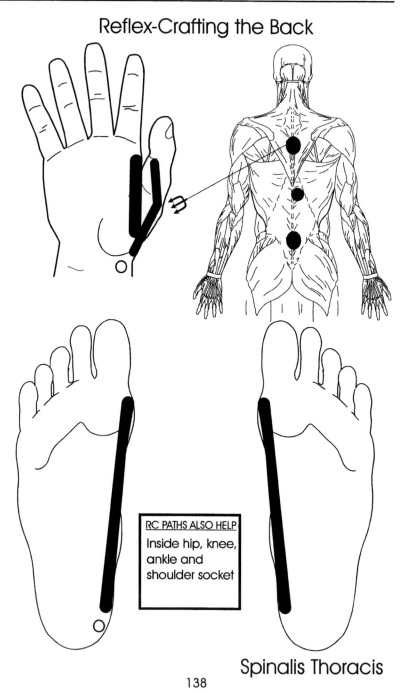

RC PATHS ALSO HELP

Inside hip, knee, ankle and shoulder socket

Spinalis Thoracis

138

Reflex-Crafting the Back

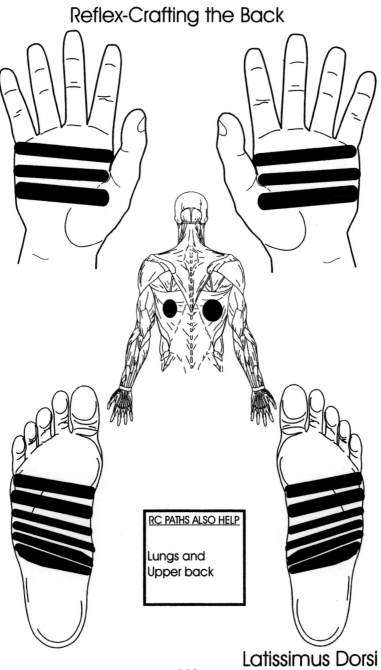

RC PATHS ALSO HELP

Lungs and
Upper back

Latissimus Dorsi

Reflex-Crafting the Back

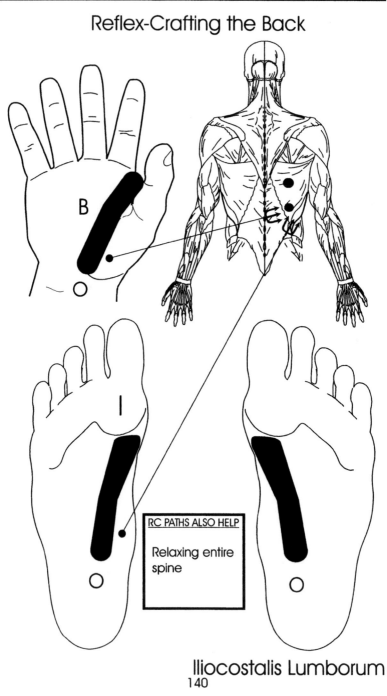

B

I

RC PATHS ALSO HELP

Relaxing entire spine

Iliocostalis Lumborum

Reflex-Crafting the Rotator Cuff

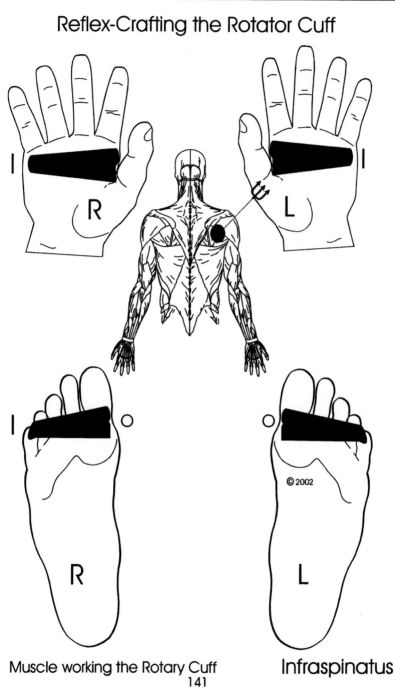

Muscle working the Rotary Cuff

Infraspinatus

141

Reflex-Crafting the Shoulder

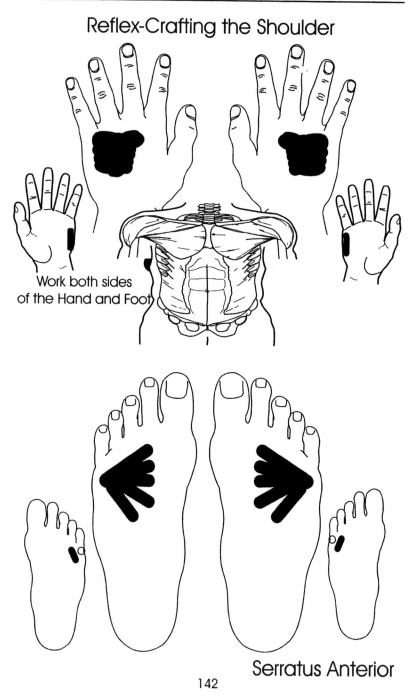

Work both sides
of the Hand and Foot

Serratus Anterior

Reflex-Crafting the Anterior Neck

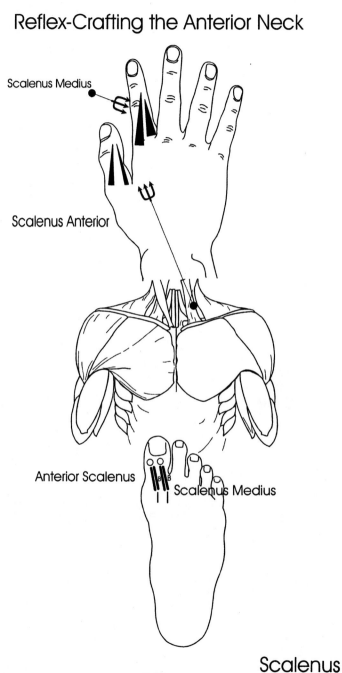

Scalenus Medius

Scalenus Anterior

Anterior Scalenus

Scalenus Medius

Scalenus

Reflex-Crafting the Torso

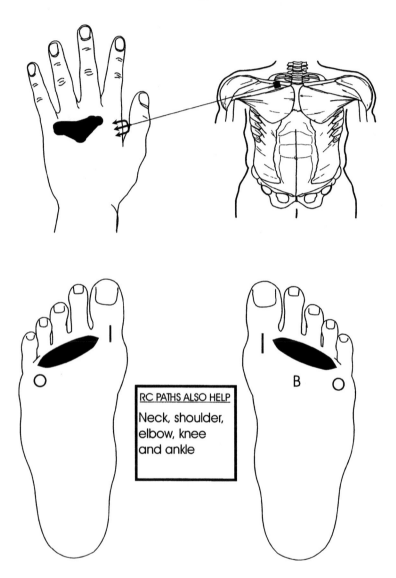

RC PATHS ALSO HELP

Neck, shoulder,
elbow, knee
and ankle

Clavicle

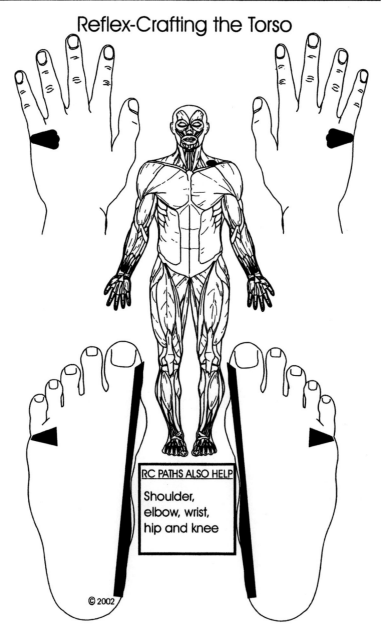

Reflex-Crafting the Torso

RC PATHS ALSO HELP

Shoulder,
elbow, wrist,
hip and knee

© 2002

Subscapularis

Reflex-Crafting the Torso

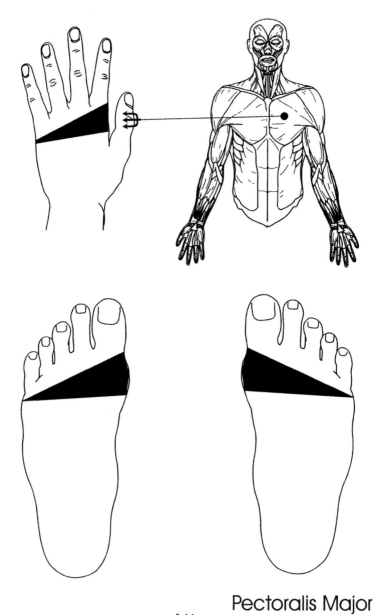

Pectoralis Major

Reflex-Crafting the Torso

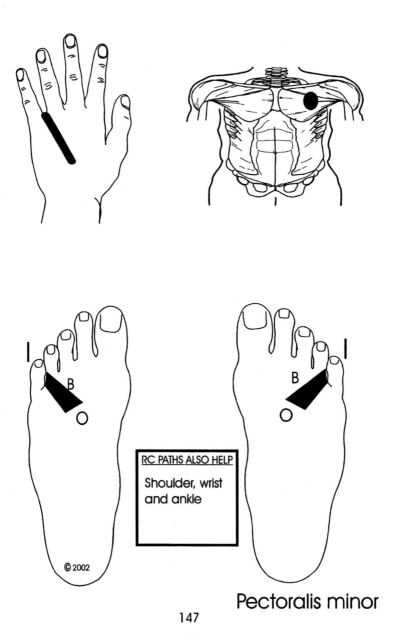

I
B
O

I
B
O

RC PATHS ALSO HELP

Shoulder, wrist
and ankle

© 2002

Pectoralis minor

Reflex-Crafting the Neck and Torso

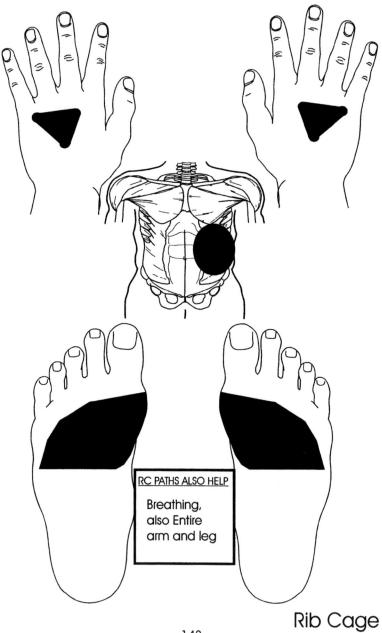

RC PATHS ALSO HELP

Breathing,
also Entire
arm and leg

Rib Cage

Reflex-Crafting the Neck and Torso

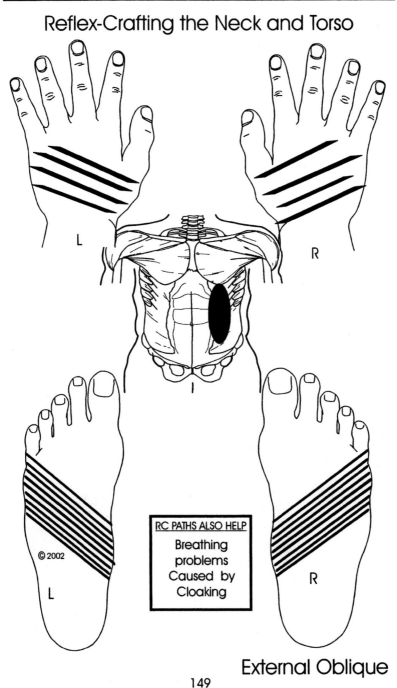

L

R

RC PATHS ALSO HELP
Breathing
problems
Caused by
Cloaking

© 2002

L

R

External Oblique

Reflex-Crafting the Torso

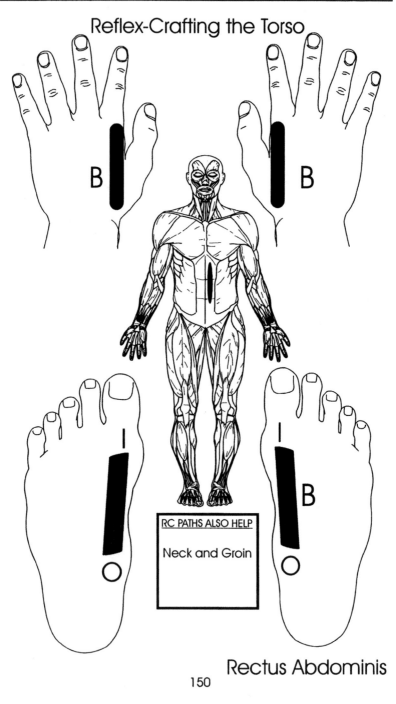

B

B

B

RC PATHS ALSO HELP

Neck and Groin

Rectus Abdominis

Reflex-Crafting the Torso

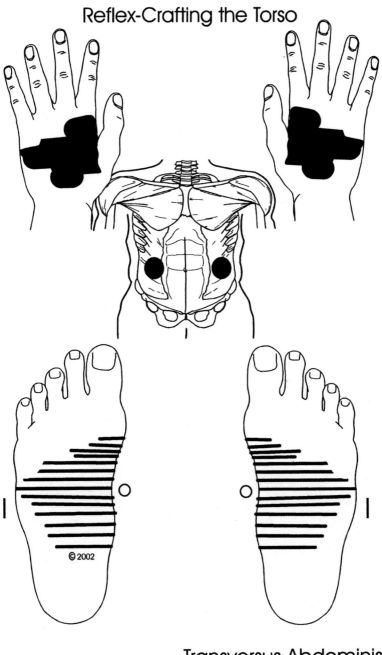

© 2002

Transversus Abdominis

151

Reflex-Crafting the Torso

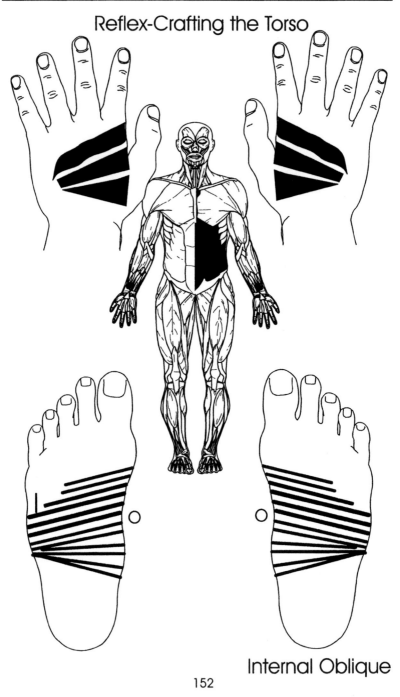

Internal Oblique

Reflex-Crafting the Torso

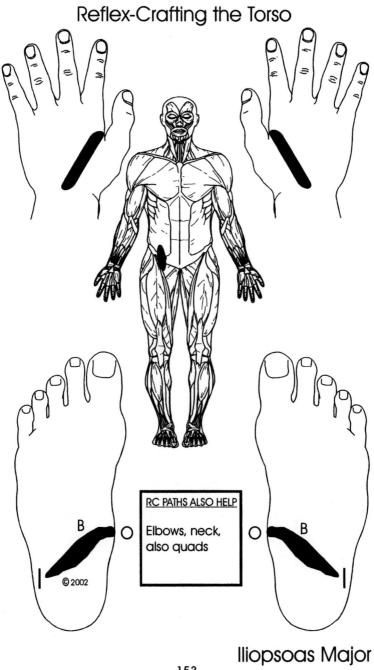

RC PATHS ALSO HELP

Elbows, neck,
also quads

B

I

© 2002

Iliopsoas Major

153

Arm, Wrist and Elbow

Use RC Sedative Crushing and Sedative Pinching
on the Hands, Feet and <u>Body</u>

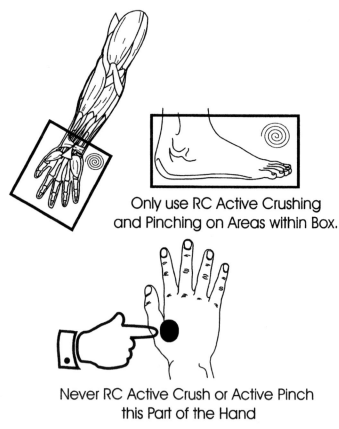

Only use RC Active Crushing
and Pinching on Areas within Box.

Never RC Active Crush or Active Pinch
this Part of the Hand

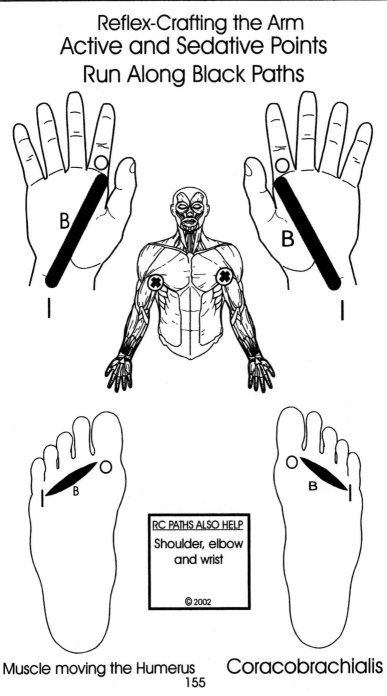

Reflex-Crafting the Arm
Active and Sedative Points
Run Along Black Paths

B

I

B

I

B

I

O

B

I

RC PATHS ALSO HELP

Shoulder, elbow
and wrist

© 2002

Muscle moving the Humerus   Coracobrachialis

Reflex-Crafting the Arm

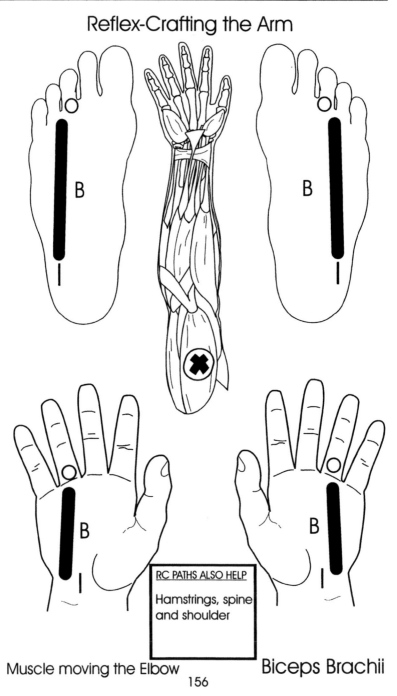

RC PATHS ALSO HELP

Hamstrings, spine and shoulder

Muscle moving the Elbow

Biceps Brachii

156

Reflex-Crafting the Arm

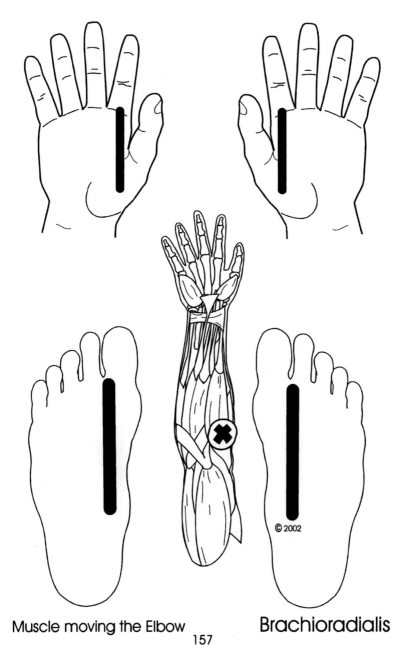

Muscle moving the Elbow

Brachioradialis

© 2002

Reflex-Crafting the Arm

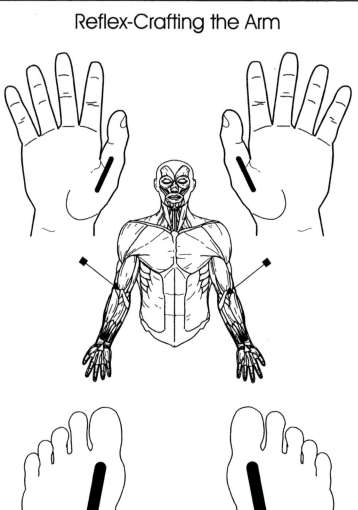

Muscle moving the Elbow   Brachialis

Reflex-Crafting the Arm

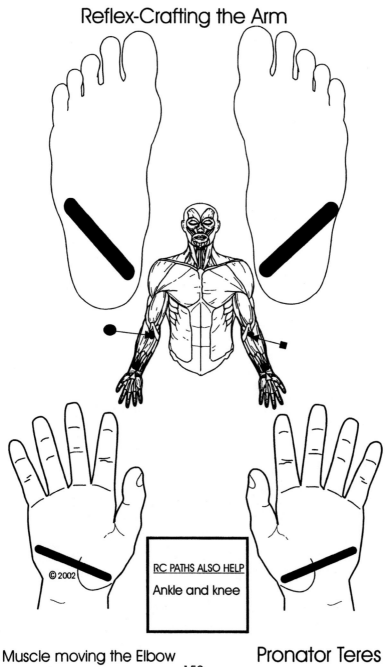

© 2002

RC PATHS ALSO HELP

Ankle and knee

Muscle moving the Elbow

Pronator Teres

159

Reflex-Crafting the Arm

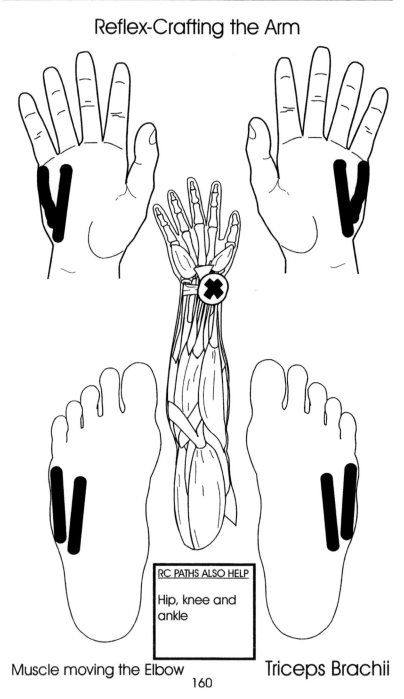

RC PATHS ALSO HELP

Hip, knee and
ankle

Muscle moving the Elbow

Triceps Brachii

Reflex-Crafting the Arm

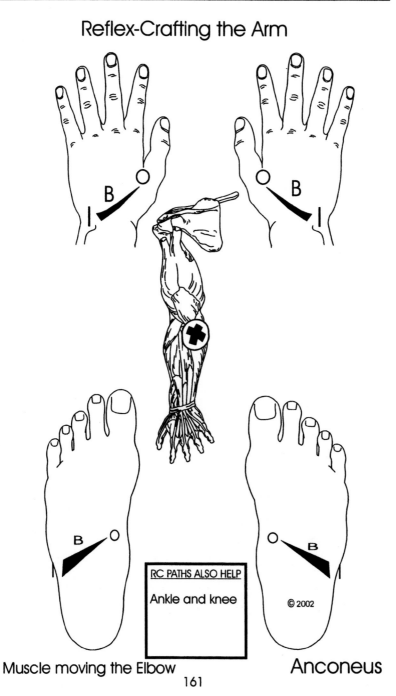

RC PATHS ALSO HELP

Ankle and knee

© 2002

Muscle moving the Elbow

Anconeus

161

Reflex-Crafting the Arm

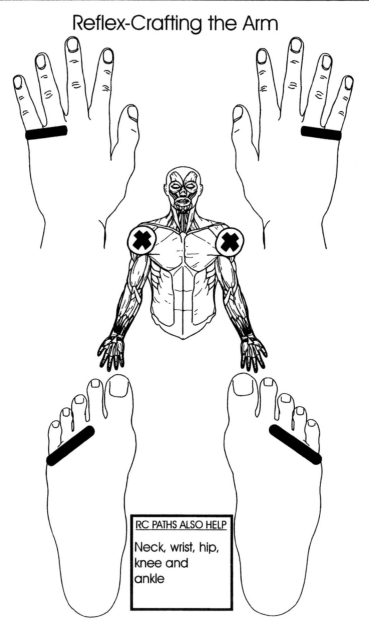

RC PATHS ALSO HELP
Neck, wrist, hip, knee and ankle

Muscle moving the Humerus

162

Deltoids

Reflex-Crafting the Arm

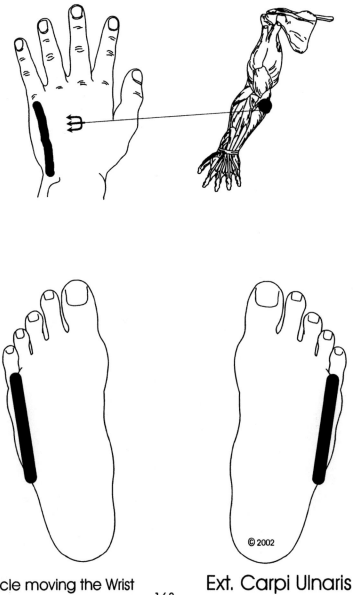

Muscle moving the Wrist

Ext. Carpi Ulnaris

© 2002

163

Reflex-Crafting the Arm

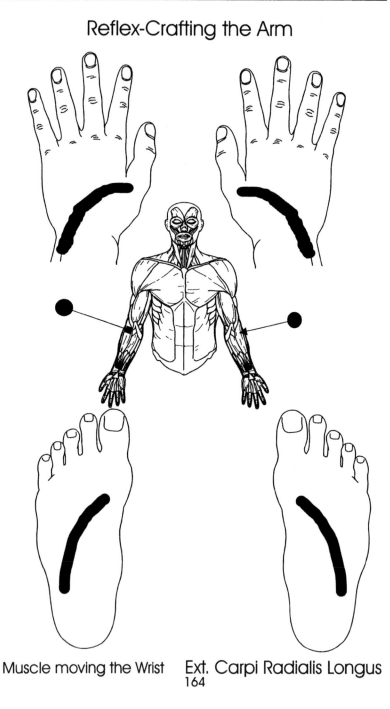

Muscle moving the Wrist   Ext. Carpi Radialis Longus

Reflex-Crafting the Arm

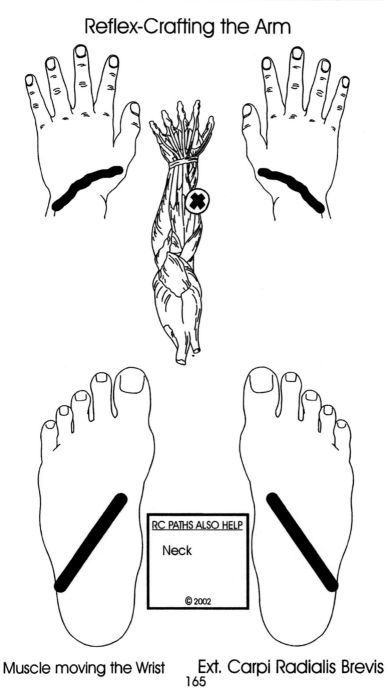

RC PATHS ALSO HELP

Neck

© 2002

Muscle moving the Wrist   Ext. Carpi Radialis Brevis

Reflex-Crafting the Arm

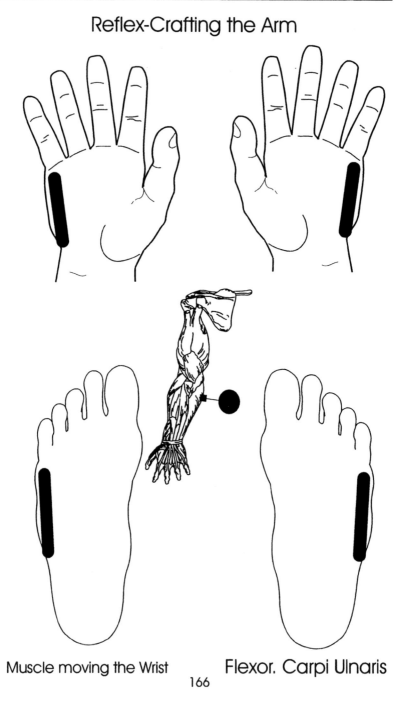

Muscle moving the Wrist   Flexor. Carpi Ulnaris

Reflex-Crafting the Arm

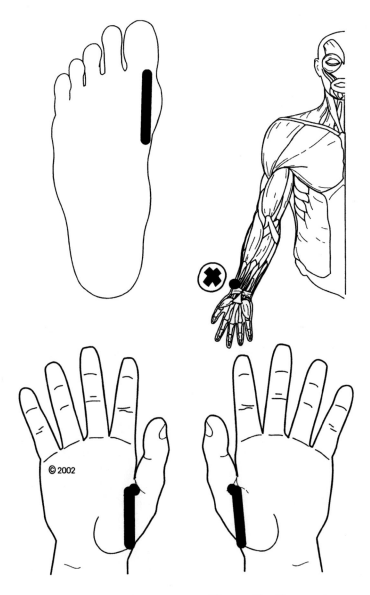

© 2002

Muscle moving the Wrist   **Flex. Pollicus Longus**

Reflex-Crafting the Arm

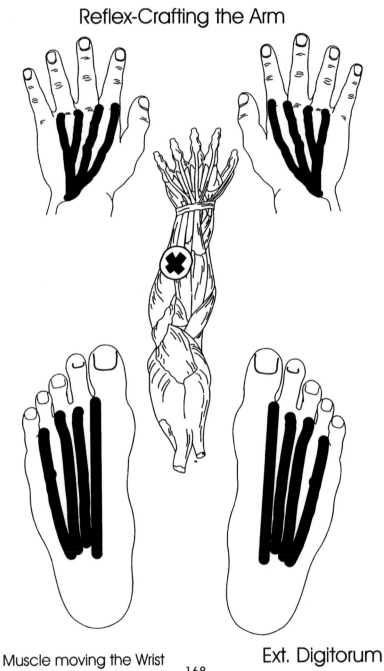

Muscle moving the Wrist

Ext. Digitorum

Reflex-Crafting the Arm

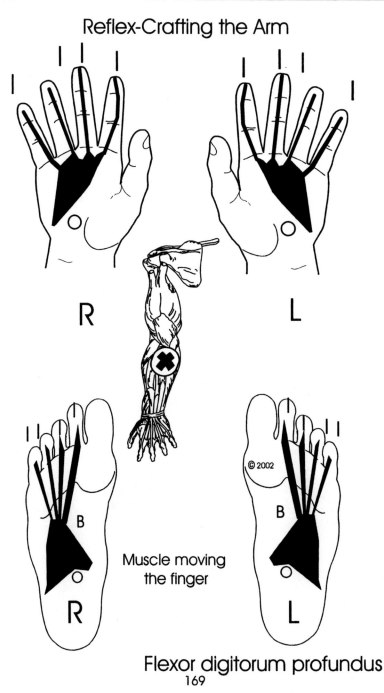

Muscle moving
the finger

Flexor digitorum profundus

Reflex-Crafting the Arm

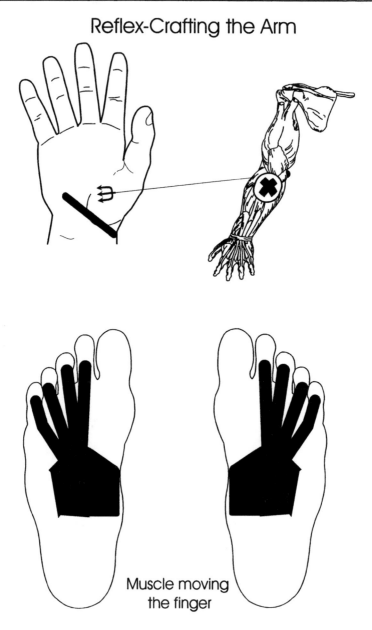

Muscle moving
the finger

Flex. Digitorum Superficialis

Reflex-Crafting the Arm

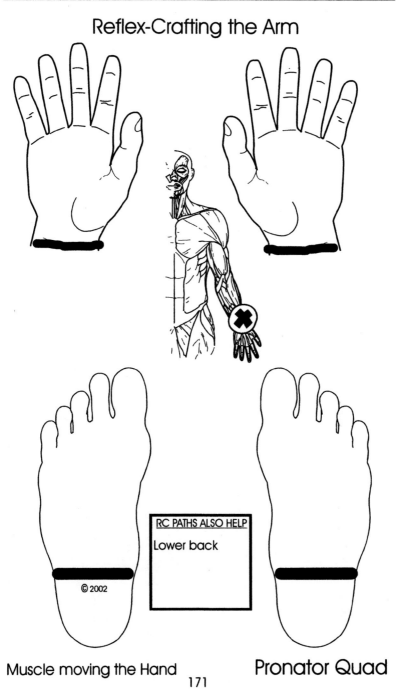

RC PATHS ALSO HELP

Lower back

© 2002

Muscle moving the Hand

Pronator Quad

171

Reflex-Crafting the Arm

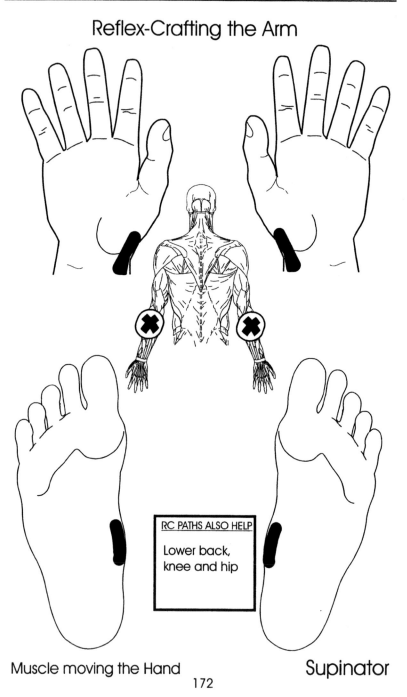

RC PATHS ALSO HELP

Lower back,
knee and hip

Muscle moving the Hand

Supinator

172

Reflex-Crafting the Arm

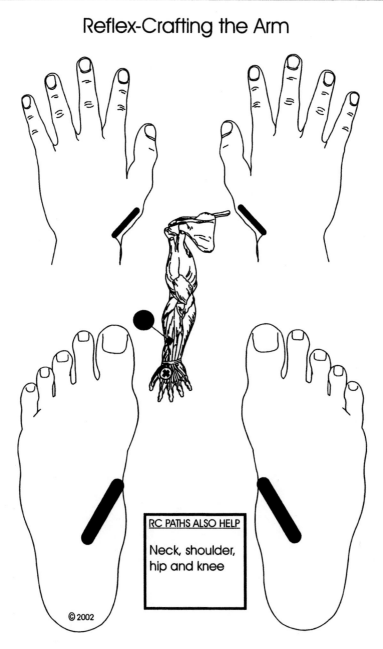

RC PATHS ALSO HELP

Neck, shoulder, hip and knee

© 2002

Muscle moving the Thumb   Abd. Pollicis Longus

Reflex-Crafting the Arm

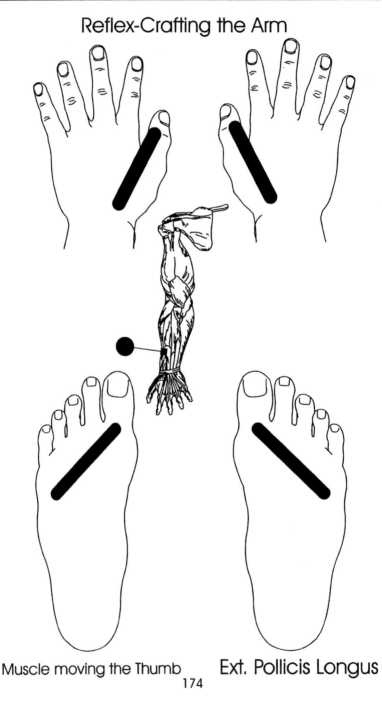

Muscle moving the Thumb   Ext. Pollicis Longus

Reflex-Crafting the Arm

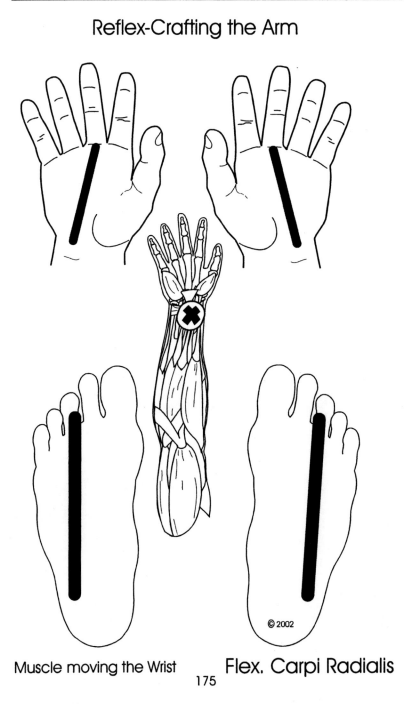

© 2002

Muscle moving the Wrist   **Flex. Carpi Radialis**

Reflex-Crafting the Arm

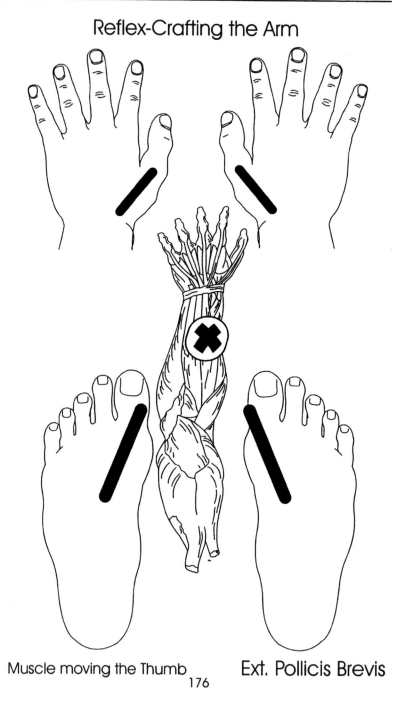

Muscle moving the Thumb

Ext. Pollicis Brevis

Upper and Lower Leg and the Knee

Reflex-Crafting Adductors

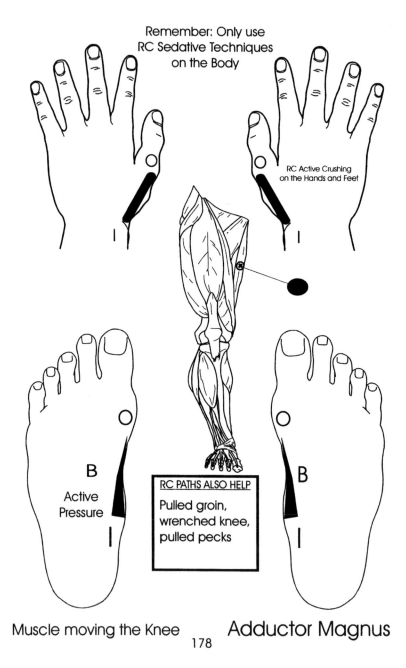

Remember: Only use
RC Sedative Techniques
on the Body

RC Active Crushing
on the Hands and Feet

B
Active
Pressure

RC PATHS ALSO HELP

Pulled groin,
wrenched knee,
pulled pecks

B

Muscle moving the Knee

Adductor Magnus

Reflex-Crafting Adductors

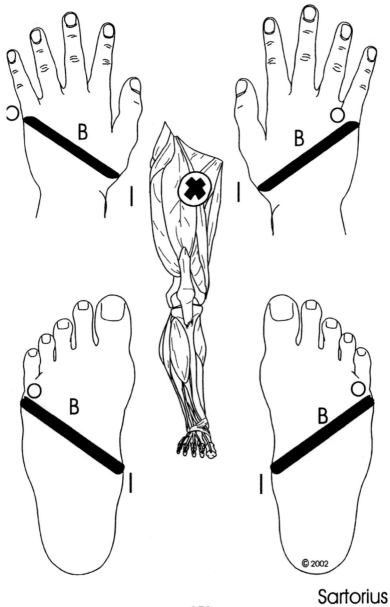

B

I   I

B

B

B

I   I

© 2002

Sartorius

179

Reflex-Crafting Adductors

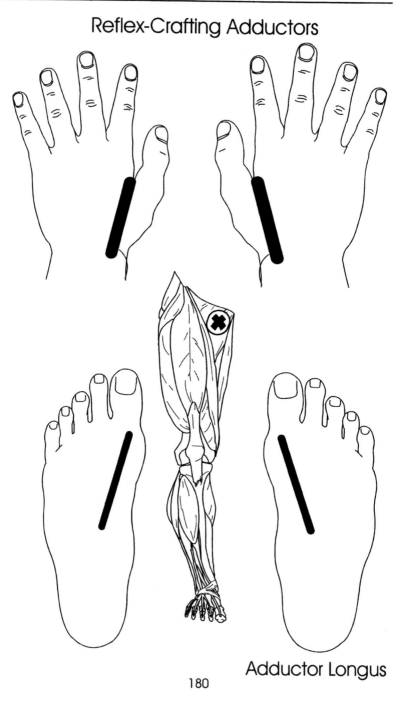

Adductor Longus

Reflex-Crafting Adductors

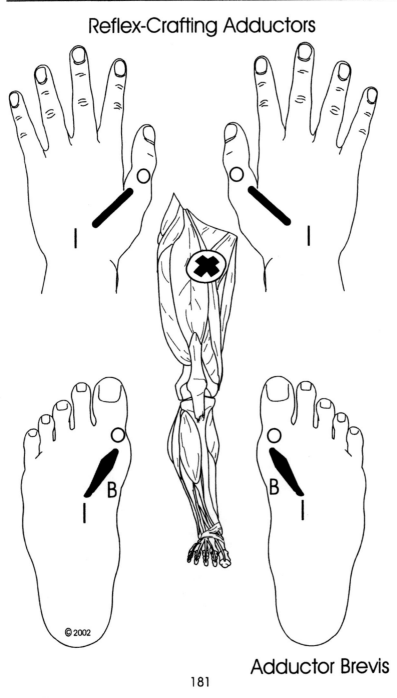

© 2002

Adductor Brevis

Reflex-Crafting Adductors

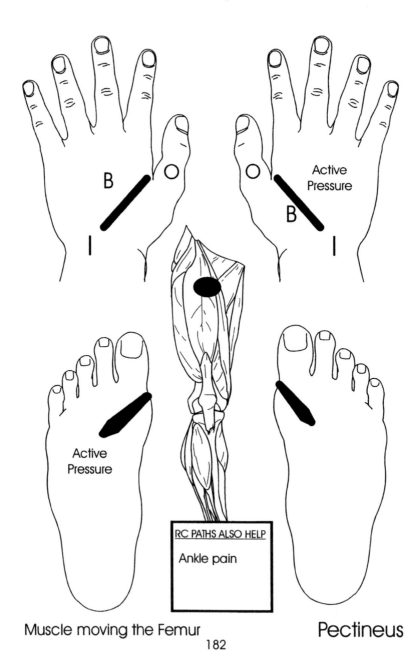

B

O

Active
Pressure

O

B

I

I

Active
Pressure

RC PATHS ALSO HELP

Ankle pain

Muscle moving the Femur

Pectineus

Reflex-Crafting Adductors

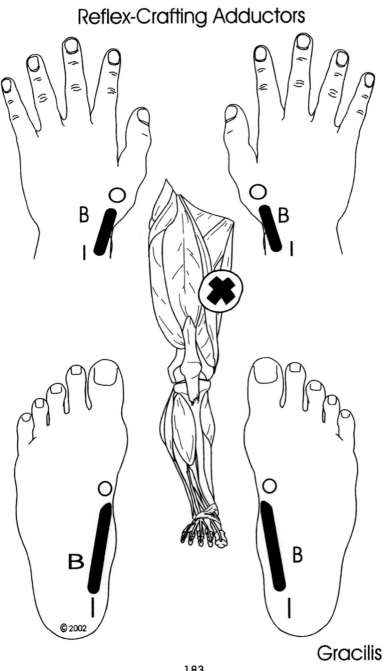

© 2002

Gracilis

Reflex-Crafting the Quadriceps

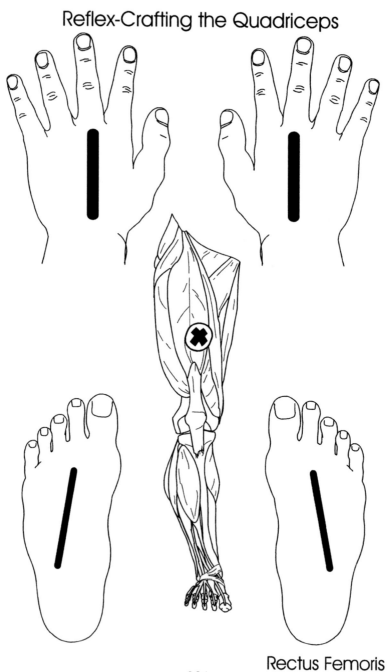

Rectus Femoris

Reflex-Crafting the Quadriceps

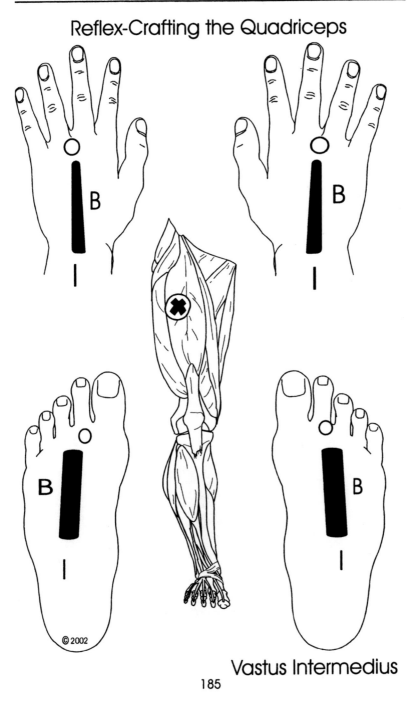

© 2002

Vastus Intermedius

Reflex-Crafting the Quadriceps

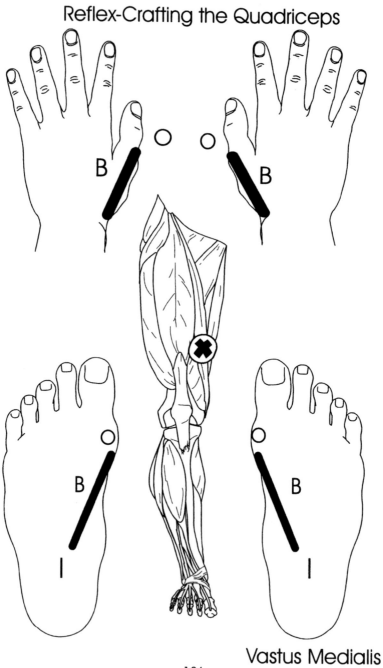

Vastus Medialis

Reflex-Crafting the Quadriceps

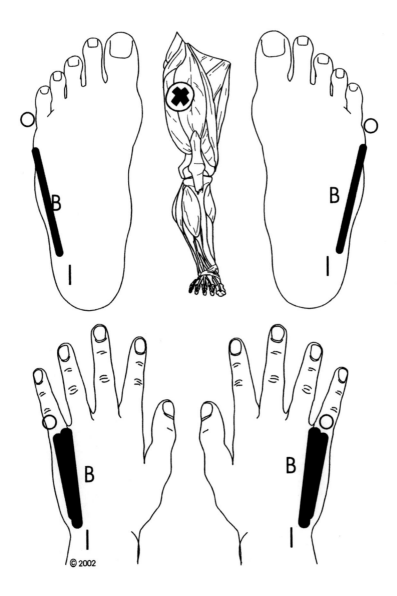

© 2002

Muscle moving the Knee

Vastus Lateralis

Reflex-Crafting the Knee

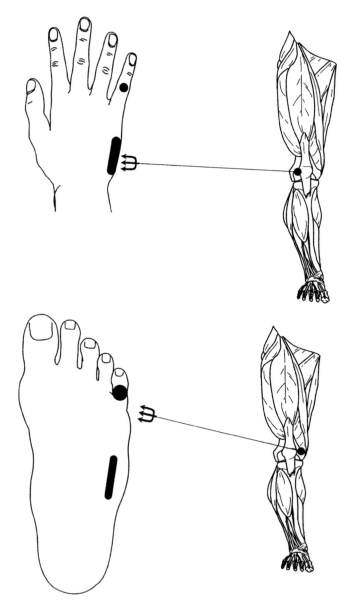

Knee

Reflex-Crafting the Knee

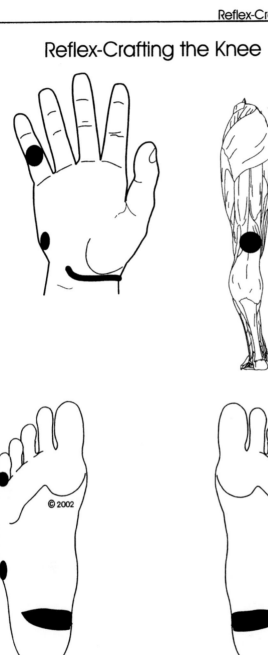

© 2002

Knee (Posterior)

Reflex-Crafting the Lower Leg

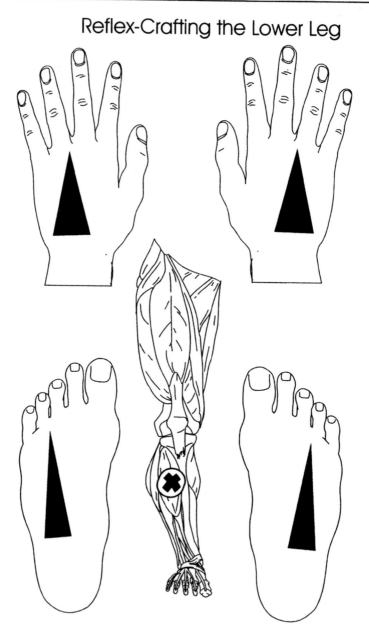

Extensor Digitorum Longus

Reflex-Crafting the Lower Leg

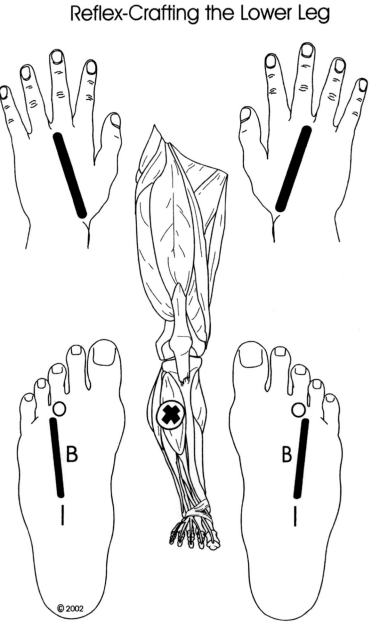

B
I

B
I

© 2002

Tibiallis Anterior

Reflex-Crafting the Lower Leg

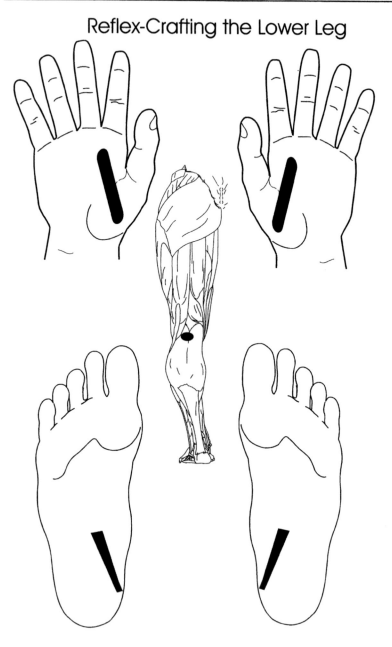

Muscle moving the Foot

Tibialis Posterior

Reflex-Crafting the Lower Leg

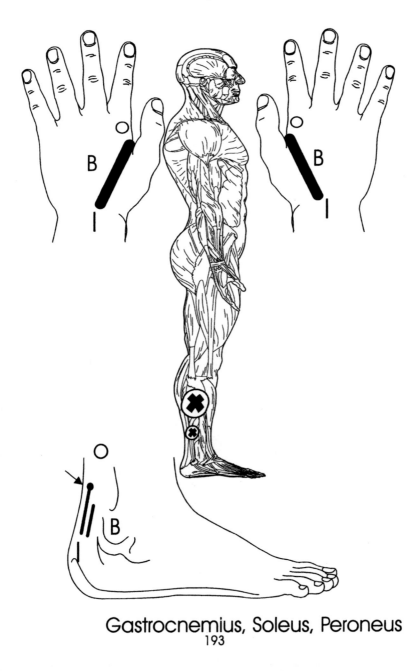

Gastrocnemius, Soleus, Peroneus

Reflex-Crafing the Upper Leg

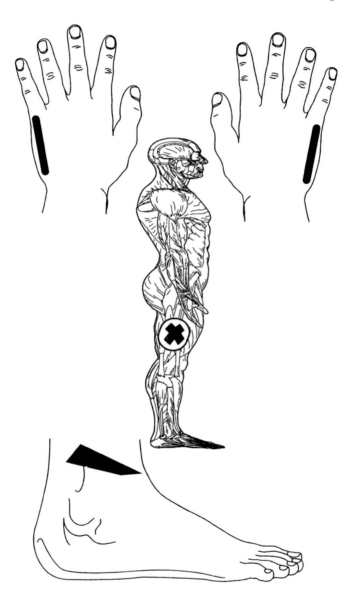

Muscle moving the Femur   Tensor Fascia Latae

Reflex-Crafting the Hip

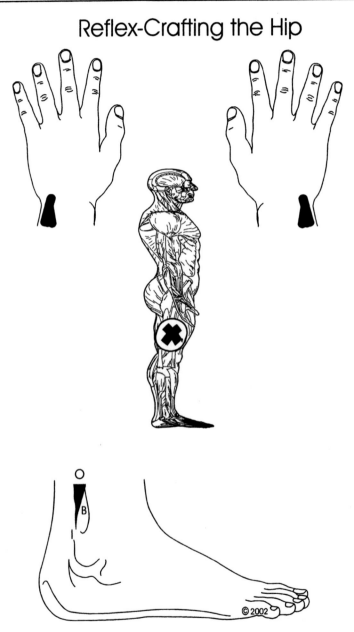

© 2002

Iliotibal Band

Reflex-Crafting the Hip and Butt

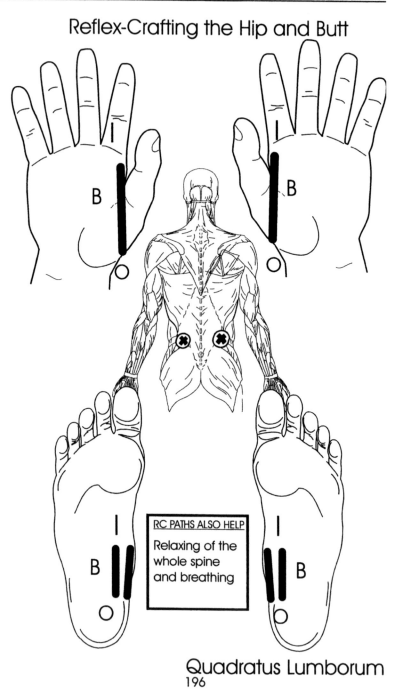

RC PATHS ALSO HELP

Relaxing of the whole spine and breathing

Quadratus Lumborum
196

Reflex-Crafting the Hip and Butt

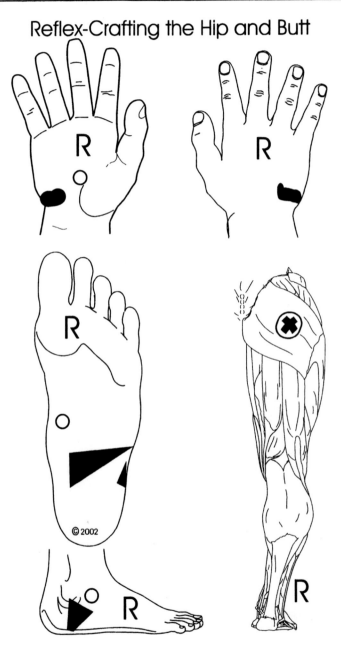

© 2002

Gluteus Minimus

Reflex-Crafting the Hip and Butt

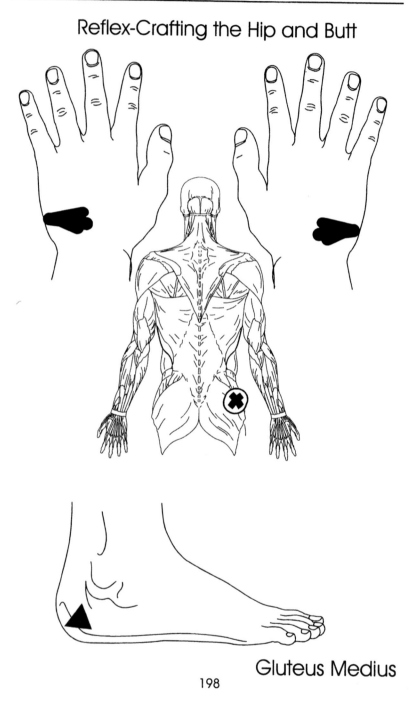

Gluteus Medius

Reflex-Crafting the Hip and Butt

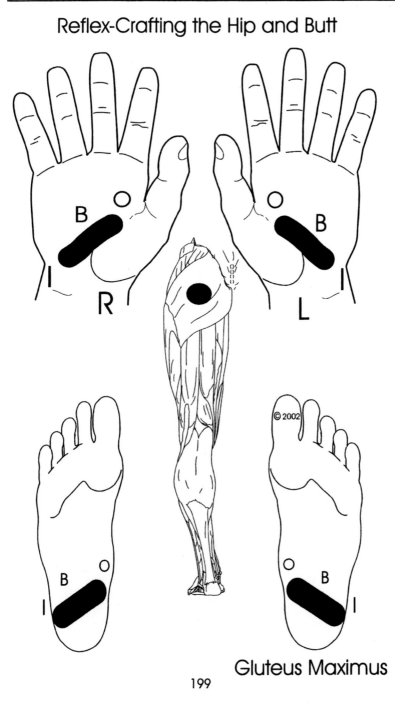

© 2002

Gluteus Maximus

Reflex-Crafting the Hip and Butt

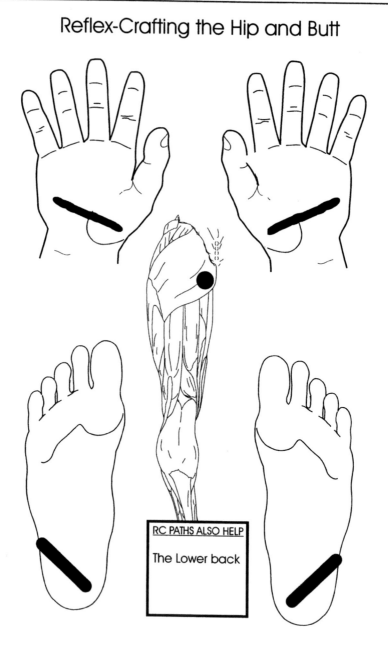

RC PATHS ALSO HELP

The Lower back

A Cause of Sciatica

Pirifomis

Reflex-Crafting the Hamstrings

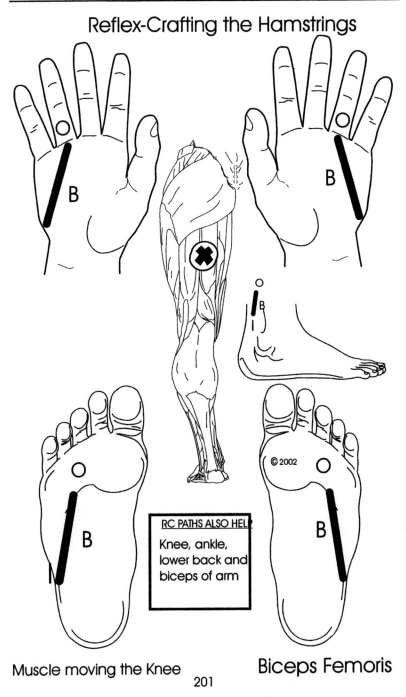

RC PATHS ALSO HELP

Knee, ankle, lower back and biceps of arm

© 2002

Muscle moving the Knee

Biceps Femoris

201

Reflex-Crafting the Hamstrings

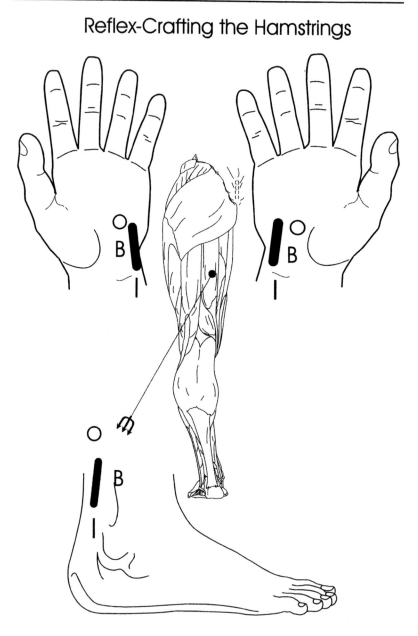

Semitendinosus

Reflex-Crafting the Hamstrings

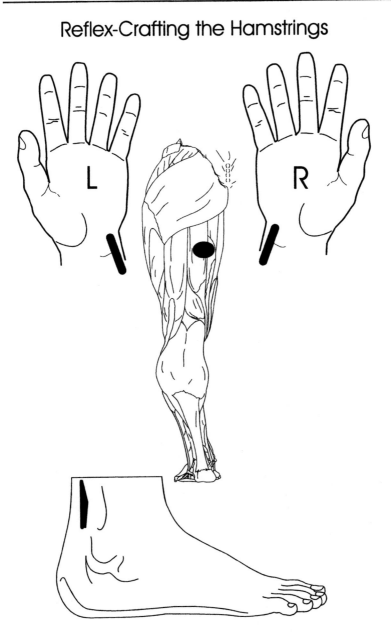

Semimembranosus

RC Guideline

Negative energy stimulates people
to push you into the fifth ring.
Anything outside the norms of the tribe,
such as being too old, too slow, too loud,
too quiet, grossly overweight or underweight
stimulates others to push.
Whereas, positive energy keeps you
in the inner rings.
Loving one another with positive thoughts
and deeds keeps all of us safe.

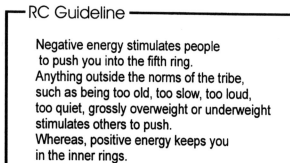

Acknowledgments

We wish to acknowledge the following companies and people for their inspiration, help and encouragement in the writing of this book.

Corel Corporation for their graphics
Lippincott Williams & Wilkins, medical art
Will Rhett and Diane Shabazian for their instruction
Marsha, Mary, Tracy and John at Hirudaya Holistic Life Center for testing the technique.
Jack and Elaine La Lanne, for their kindness
National Geographic
Animal Planet
Andrew Biel, Trail Guide to The Body
Mary Lee Morgan, our wonderful editor
Kelly LeBrock
Ed and Bobbi Davis
Artie Shaw, King of Swing
Ellarae Markhart
Tom and Beth Majors
Milton Bilak, Dorian Francis Bilak
Dr. Fanya Carter
Art Tilton
Rick Crane
Karen Grencik
Sally DeVine
Kathy Johnson
Kay Pick
Sara Loven
Bruce Clendenen
Don and Johanna Vokal
Bev Zastoupil
Carolyn Mueller and Gordon Peterson

To Order This Book:

Please make payment in U.S. dollars of $16.95, plus shipping/handling of $3.05, for a total of $20.00 per book. California residents add appropriate sales tax. Prices and availability are subject to change at any time without notice.

Send this order form with your check to:
Reflex-Crafting, P.O. Box 6676, Los Osos, California 93412. Allow 4-6 weeks for delivery.

SHIP TO:
Name: _____
Address: _____
City/State/Zip: _____
Telephone: _____